If you've picked up this book, you're probably worried about your child—things just don't seem "right." This comprehensive guide enables parents, children, and their doctor to identify and treat this often-difficult-to-diagnose disease. Know the facts:

- The younger the child is when he or she develops fibromyalgia, the more likely it is that both parents have fibromyalgia.

- A diagnosis of attention-deficit disorder could be a red flag for fibromyalgia.

- While there is an equal proportion of boys and girls suffering from pediatric fibromyalgia, most boys will outgrow the disease after puberty.

- After children attain most of their adult height and weight, the danger of fibromyalgia, at least for girls, becomes progressively greater with each passing year.

- It's crucial to find a physician, massage therapist, physical therapist, or chiropractor to examine and "map" your child before starting guaifenesin.

- An observant parent can identify the disease and get treatment for a child before symptoms become debilitating.

IF YOU SUSPECT YOUR CHILD IS SUFFERING FROM THIS DEVASTATING DISEASE, IT'S TIME TO LEARN ...

WHAT YOUR DOCTOR MAY *NOT* TELL YOU ABOUT
PEDIATRIC
FIBROMYALGIA

WHAT YOUR DOCTOR MAY *NOT* TELL YOU ABOUT PEDIATRIC FIBROMYALGIA

A Safe New Treatment Plan for Children

R. PAUL ST. AMAND, M.D. and CLAUDIA CRAIG MAREK

WARNER BOOKS

An AOL Time Warner Company

The information herein is not intended to replace the services of trained health professionals, or be a substitute for medical advice. You are advised to consult with your health care professional with regard to matters relating to your health, and in particular regarding matters that may require diagnosis or medical attention.

The title of the series What Your Doctor May *Not* Tell You about . . . and the related trade dress are trademarks owned by Warner Books, Inc., and may not be used without permission.

Warner Books, Inc., 1271 Avenue of the Americas, New York, NY 10020
Visit our Web site at www.twbookmark.com.

 An AOL Time Warner Company

Printed in the United States of America
First Printing: November 2002
10 9 8 7 6 5 4 3 2 1

Library of Congress Cataloging-in-Publication Data

St. Amand, R. Paul
    What your doctor may not tell you about pediatric fibromyalgia : a safe, new treatment plan for children / R. Paul St. Amand, and Claudia Craig Marek.
        p. cm.
    Includes index.
    ISBN 0-446-67994-1
    1. Fibromyalgia. 2. Fibromyalgia—Treatment. 3. Children—Diseases—Treatment. I. Marek, Claudia. II. Title.

RC927.3 .S733 2002
618.92'74—dc21   2002069132

Book design by Charles Sutherland
Cover design by Diane Luger

Acknowledgments

Each and every book written owes debts to many contributors both direct and indirect—and this one is no exception. First of all, we must thank our families for their understanding about the demands this project made upon our time. Our children (and now grandchildren!) who have fibromyalgia have been our laboratories and our inspiration and have graciously allowed us to use their stories. Malcolm Potter, who has grown up from the little boy on the first page of this book to working in our office, is now helping others cope with this devastating illness. Malcolm was our first patient on guaifenesin, and to him we are especially grateful.

This book also owes much to Gloria Martinez, who worked daily compiling statistics and running the office. Without her this task would have been immensely more difficult, and less complete. This small paragraph can't begin to convey the depth of our appreciation for eighteen years of loyal and loving support.

Jessica Papain and Diana Baroni, our editors, have worked many hours teaching and supporting us, and we also owe them a large debt of gratitude. Carol Mann, our agent, has guided us and advised us with wisdom and patience from the beginning.

Finally, as always, we must thank our patients, and our correspondents for the use of their observations and quotations, and for their support. Tesa Marcon, owner of the guai-support group on the Internet, Gwen Meshorer, and Jeri Dutcher stand out as others who should be given a special thank-you. Our work and our protocol owe much to the tireless efforts of many around the world, and we are in debt to each and every one of them.

Contents

Preface

One evening in the Lake Country of England, where I stayed recently on vacation, I leaned against a fence, mesmerized, watching some of the sheep that dotted the landscape. Among them were six lambs, five gathered on the opposite side of the field from a single one. As I stood and watched, the quintet would suddenly dash off with a speed I never thought possible for lambs. They would leap into the air almost in unison, arching their backs with Olympic-quality gymnastic moves. Each time they passed me, the same lamb led, with the other four maintaining the same file position. A few times they ran to the side of the lone lamb, who only then would join the pack. But each time she did, she would stop after just a few leaps and then simply stand and watch the group continue its woolly ballet, unable or unwilling to follow.

If we are observant, the spectrum of youthful behavior readily unfolds for us. In my forty-four years in clinical practice I have seen many children with fibromyalgia. I thought of them as I observed the lambs. Children seem to settle early into certain posi-

tions within their childhood society—often the ones to which they will gravitate throughout their lives. Are there those who could—and should—be leading but who never quite achieve their potential? Like my little lamb that just could not play as the other lambs were doing—are these children on the sidelines for reasons they do not understand?

First, I extend a disclaimer. I am not a pediatrician, and as a rule, I do not treat children. In the past, I rarely accepted pediatric endocrinology cases. I felt that these problems were best diagnosed and treated by specialists in that intricate field. In my office we scheduled only adults, and my teaching in endocrinology these past forty-four years was always limited to that age group. In time, however, parents began discussing symptoms they had observed in their children. At their request, I began examining some of these youngsters. It was soon obvious that there was a pediatric version of fibromyalgia. This is why we are writing this book: to provide, especially for mothers, the means by which they can suspect the disease in their offspring.

My work with fibromyalgia actually began some forty years ago, when I realized I had stumbled onto a new condition, a no-name entity that affected mostly women. These patients were highly symptomatic and were commonly considered neurotic, complaining of depression, anxiety, apathy, aches and pains, headaches, and often weight gain. Contemporary conventional medical wisdom was to give these women tranquilizers to "settle their nerves." But nearly from the beginning I was convinced that their illness had a metabolic cause. I just could not accept that so many women had complaints solely of psychiatric origin. A little later on, I found that certain medications, normally reserved for the treatment of gout, were highly effective at reversing this supposedly nonexistent disease.

By the time the multiple and scattered complaints of this disease were finally linked and officially designated "fibromyalgia," I had already treated hundreds of patients successfully. Many people knew that I had this head start and spread the word. My success in reversing the newly identified syndrome drew more patients to my office.

Soon my practice consisted mainly of women simply because 85 percent of fibromyalgics are female. Many of them are mothers and, obviously, of the 15 percent who are males, many are fathers. These parents frequently discussed the symptoms displayed by their children, usually daughters. These complaints had jostled memories of their own childhood. In the end, these observations were repeated by so many parents that I began to realize there was such an illness as pediatric fibromyalgia. Since there has to be a beginning to all illnesses, what were the earliest symptoms of fibromyalgia? There would probably be only an occult few and they would be difficult to analyze. When my own daughters developed some of the telltale complaints and tissue swellings, I quickly became more than casually interested. All three showed obvious symptoms and findings by the respective ages of eleven, thirteen, and sixteen. I was chagrined to realize that I had passed my defective gene(s) on to my daughters as my father had to me. As I listened more attentively to parental concerns and observations, we came to realize the prevalence and severity of fibromyalgia in children. For these compelling reasons, it seemed mandatory that we write this book.

I have frequently seen gifted children, former achievers, gradually succumb to some braking force. Their behavior seems to deteriorate into a mixture of fatigue, erratic emotions, and apathy—totally uncharacteristic of their earlier demeanor. Parents, especially mothers, know that this is not normal for their children, and, often against great odds, seek answers. These children demonstrate no external stigma that would separate them or prevent them from blending into their peer group. Yet they are distinctly different from the others, and often from their younger selves. Their mothers, my patients, turned to me in desperation and pleaded with me to help. This is how I became involved in these children's lives, in their struggles, and eventually in their treatment.

So it was that I began accepting children into my practice, at first only the offspring of my own patients. We gradually accumulated the histories of and findings from many children under age sixteen, from whom we have gathered many of the facts we will present in this book.

This book is about the different lambs, the children who are afflicted with fibromyalgia, an illness inherited from one or both parents. It is based on the few hundred we have treated, and others who have generously shared their stories with us by letter or by e-mail. It is also about fibromyalgic adults who came late to their diagnosis. Many will be reminded of their own painful childhood. They will relive their growing pains, diminished teenage endurance, and restricted athletic ability. They will recall with anguish their feelings of being unlike others and the resulting isolation. Many have gone on to productive and successful lives—often by carefully developing talents in areas where they could pace themselves, or adapt within their limitations. With extraordinary willpower and tenacity, they were able to overcome blunted cognitive abilities and merciless apathy.

I have come to know fibromyalgic children largely through the extraordinary dedication of their mothers, who ignored the doctors who tried to convince them their children were psychologically impaired, or that they were overly protective. I marvel at their stubborn refusal to accept "nothing is wrong" when "all the tests are normal." Many women instinctively suspected the diagnosis from the blight of their own fibromyalgia. My coauthor, Claudia Craig Marek, draws on her childhood experience with her own symptoms and those of her two boys. She is one of these stalwart mothers, the women to whom I dedicate this book.

R. Paul St. Amand, M.D.
Marina del Rey, California
November 2000

WHAT YOUR DOCTOR MAY *NOT* TELL YOU ABOUT

PEDIATRIC FIBROMYALGIA

Chapter 1

What Is Fibromyalgia?

It feels like every muscle in my body is going to throw up.
—*Malcolm Potter, age eight, Los Angeles, California*

I especially and clearly remember periods of extended lethargy and tiredness when I was too tired, didn't feel like doing anything, when my friends were biking and I could not keep up, or playing ball or swimming or playing tennis, which was absolutely tortuous. I was labeled as lazy—but physically I could just not keep up. . . . When I look back at my childhood, I see a child who sometimes felt okay, but who often just trudged along thinking everyone felt this way but they overcame it because they weren't lazy.
—*S.R.C., Lancaster, South Carolina*

Fibromyalgia means simply "a condition of pain in the muscles and fibers." The name was chosen to replace fibrositis about twenty years ago. The suffix "itis" implied inflammation but as

1

there is none in this disease, the old name was quickly discarded as a bad moniker. Though pain is certainly a prominent symptom of fibromyalgia, this newer name does not very adequately describe the condition either—in adults or children. For now, as we introduce and review what fibromyalgia is, we won't be concerning ourselves with the nuances that make up the subtle differences we've observed in the different age groups of sufferers. We'll leave that topic for the next chapter. For right now, let's explore fibromyalgia in more general terms.

The illness has been around for at least as long as written history, from what we can tell. It was called rheumatism, neuralgia, myalgia, and unkinder things (like hysteria and hypochondria) before modern medicine officially defined it in the 1990s. So fibromyalgia, the name we use today, is quite possibly the same age as your child! That may be why you can't trace the condition through your family tree—there was no illness by this name even a generation ago.

We previously proposed the name *dysenergism* in our first book, *What Your Doctor May* Not *Tell You about Fibromyalgia*. We did this because we think such a name would better reflect the subjective and biochemical lack of energy that is so central in the lives of those who suffer from fibromyalgia. Only a rare patient does not feel this loss of stamina. Almost all realize how very little energy they have, and how quickly it is depleted. The best research evidence to date confirms that cells throughout the body have difficulty producing energy, and corroborates what patients have been stressing. The most common recollection of adults who had symptoms as children was of the rapid waning of endurance compared to that of their peers. Pain, while a common complaint, seems to arise from tissue that can't make enough energy, and stiffness, cramping, and aching are a result of that. It's highly unlikely, of course, that the name will be changed again, but as you read along, bear in mind that the name fibromyalgia itself isn't very descriptive of the totality of this condition, which really has an effect on almost every cell of the body.

There are no blood tests, or any other standard medical tests that show any abnormalities unique to fibromyalgia, so the disease can't be diagnosed the way most conditions are. Instead, if a physician suspects you or your child has the illness, there are several criteria he or she will use to confirm the diagnosis. These were first put together by a group called the American College of Rheumatology in the late 1980s. The acronym for this august body (ACR) is one you'll surely come across a lot if you do any reading in medical journals.

Although we don't use the ACR criteria in our practice, per se, we think we should let you know what they are. The reason for this is that most doctors do use what we consider this overly narrow view of the illness. Most of what you read is based on this original work.

So what is the textbook description of fibromyalgia according to the "official party line" of the World Health Organization, the gospel according to the ACR that was delivered via the World Congress in Copenhagen in 1992? Well, fibromyalgia is defined first and foremost as a painful condition of muscles that causes chronic and widespread pain or aching throughout the whole body—that is, in all four quadrants of the body, for more than four months' duration. This pain or aching is qualified by the word "unexplained," meaning that it has no known cause, such as being run over by a truck.

Though you may feel as if you've been run over by road-building equipment in the mornings when you wake up, if you actually have been, then you have pain but not fibromyalgia! Next you must have some of the other symptoms: morning stiffness and nonrestorative sleep, and the presence of tender points—that is, tenderness in eleven of eighteen predetermined sites. Headaches, irritable bladder, restless legs, insomnia, exercise intolerance, weakness, areas of abnormal sensations such as numbness, tingling, and cold extremities round out the list of "official complaints."

As you'll read below, we examine the whole body for abnormal findings, not just a few spots. We also record and monitor quite a few more symptoms, some of which, admittedly, are accepted as part of fibromyalgia now, but were not mentioned back in 1990. The ensuing years have brought forth some newly accepted relationships between fibromyalgia and other symptoms, such as vulvodynia, skin sensations, and increased sensitivities to chemicals, sound, and noise.

Fibromyalgia is known to affect mostly women, about 85 percent of those diagnosed. It's not as uncommon as you might think: Statistics show at least 5 percent of the population probably has it, and about 20 percent of patients seen by rheumatologists are eventually told that they have the illness.

Most books and papers about fibromyalgia repeat as a litany that it presents mainly between the ages of twenty-five and fifty-five. Yet we know that it can manifest itself in any year of life. We have seen patients with disease onset as young as two and as old as seventy-four. Had these authors been involved in treating the full spectrum of patients and the illness, they would have better recognized its frequency in all age groups. Should they not wonder what has happened to patients over fifty-five? Similarly, should they not ask themselves when does fibromyalgia first begin and what are its earliest symptoms? It can be easily seen from looking at the original defining papers on fibromyalgia that nowhere is it stated that patients must be over or under a certain age. It was only later papers, studying the demographics of the illness, that gave rise to this now too-commonly held belief. Some physicians will staunchly insist fibromyalgia can't exist in children or men. When it comes to the latter, they'll often call the condition "chronic fatigue syndrome" despite the fact that patients may also complain of chronic pain or stiffness.

Pain is certainly an important clue used in making the diagnosis of fibromyalgia. It's rare to encounter a patient with no pain, but pain is subjective, and we've noticed that most people really don't consider it their primary complaint. Exhaustion, fatigue, and poor stamina are usually listed first. Children may also complain of fatigue and irritable bowel symptoms more often than, say, shoulder pain. Older patients may be troubled by depression and sleep disturbances. That's why it's important for us to stop for a minute and examine all the common symptoms of this disease.

The full-blown picture of fibromyalgia is overwhelming because so many bodily structures and systems are affected by diminished energy production. For clarification only, we usually separate the symptoms into groups we call syndromes. However, the head bone *is* connected to the toe bone. The interlocking biochemistry and physiology of living tissues mandates a strong interplay between all the body's systems, however separate they may seem.

CENTRAL NERVOUS SYSTEM

In this listing we include the so-called "brain symptoms" of fatigue, irritability, nervousness, depression, apathy, listlessness, anxieties, suicidal thoughts, and impaired memory and concentration. Insomnia can prevent one from getting to sleep even when one is exhausted. Patients cannot find a position that remains comfortable very long. Frequent awakening is common because of discomfort and pain. Consequently, sleep is rarely restful and is said to be nonrestorative.

MUSCULOSKELETAL

Pain in any muscle, tendon, ligament, or fascia may be involved, though the shoulders, neck, upper and lower back, hips, knees, inner and outer elbows, wrists, and chest are the most commonly affected. Generalized morning aching and stiffness are usually present. It is frequently stated that joints are not affected in fibromyalgia, but everyone with the disease knows better. Sites of previous injuries, either traumatic or surgical, are among the structures most involved.

IRRITABLE BOWEL

This is often called by other names, such as leaky gut, spastic colon, or mucous colitis. There is sometimes a steady abdominal aching that is probably due to the involvement of deep intra-abdominal tissues. Overacidity may cause burning in the pit of the stomach, or an acid reflux produces a burning chest pain. Nausea occurs in brief but repetitive waves. Gas and bloating create a wandering discomfort and, at times, cramping or sharp, stabbing pains. There are brief of prolonged bouts of constipation alternating with diarrhea, with or without mucus that may accompany either one.

GENITOURINARY

Increased frequency of urination is sometimes accompanied by pain in the lowest part of the abdomen caused by bladder spasms. Unrelenting pain above the pubic bone and frequent voiding, in the presence or absence of infection, evoke the diagnosis of chronic interstitial cystitis. Burning upon urination may be brief (one or two voids only) or persistent. Intermittently, urine may have a pungent odor that is difficult to describe. It smells like the breakdown product of recently ingested asparagus mixed with acid, kerosene, and new-mown hay. (Feel free to make up your own or accept that as our best description.) The vulvar pain syndrome (vulvodynia) includes deep vaginal spasms, irritation of the vaginal lips (vulvitis) or similar changes in the pelvic opening (vulvar vestibulitis). The premenstrual syndrome with uterine cramping and abdominal bloating is greatly intensified. (Everything about fibromyalgia is worse during the premenstrual week.) Vulvodynia closely mimics symptoms of yeast infections but without the usual thick, cottage-cheese discharge.

DERMATOLOGIC

Hives, red blotches, tiny bumps, blisters, eczema, seborrheic dermatitis, neurodermatitis, and acne are common. Itching occurs with or without rashes. Nails become brittle and readily peel or chip in cycles or permanently. Hair has a poor quality and falls out prematurely, often in clusters. The skin may be supersensitive to touch or to temperature changes. Sudden flushing of the ears, face, or upper front chest is frequently observed. Patients experience prickling, tingling, numbness, or burning anywhere, but especially in their palms or soles, with or without redness. Crawling sensations induce a futile search for the fallen hair or bug that is never there.

MISCELLANEOUS

Headaches are often of migraine intensity. Dizziness is mainly a sensation of imbalance, but vertigo (actual spinning) may appear in sporadic attacks. Patients often have itching, burning, or dry eyes and transient or prolonged blurring of vision. Chronic nasal congestion and postnasal drip are usually present. The entire mouth may feel as if it has been scalded, often with a metallic or foul taste. The tongue may also feel burned or scraped, especially around the edges. Swishing, flapping, or ringing (tinnitus) sounds may be heard fleetingly. Vibrations, numbness, and tingling hands, feet, or face are frightening, especially when they are accompanied by severe headaches. Leg or foot cramps are sporadic. Other symptoms occur, such as weight gain (twenty pounds or more), low-grade fevers (usually less than one hundred degrees), and increased susceptibility to infections.

Sensitivities to light, sounds, odors, or chemicals along with hay fever and asthma often lead to allergy testing. Water retention is usual during attacks and causes morning swelling of the eyelids and hands. As the day progresses, there is a gravitational shift of fluid that may induce the restless leg syndrome as the skin is stretched from within by the invisible edema.

In the end, it is often simply the sheer number of complaints that alert a physician to suspect the diagnosis. Few conditions so thoroughly invade the body. Yet, as we stated above, no abnormalities are found by the customary x-ray or laboratory studies. A few may appear with esoteric testing in research facilities but none are diagnostic of fibromyalgia. This does not mean that the illness is not real, or that it doesn't exist. It just means science hasn't figured it out yet. Any physician or other person who implies that fibromyalgia isn't a real, distinct illness isn't very well-informed. It is *not* a wastebasket, catch-all name for something that's not really accepted. It is something millions of people have, and a condition that has an effect on the lives of millions more. Too many people know too little about it, that's true. But it's not true that it isn't an accepted medical condition.

It is also true that awareness of the disease is recent, as is its sometimes abominable method of treatment. No one should so soon be allowed to steal the term "traditional" and impose a dogmatic approach to the condition, especially because so few treatments have been shown to be beneficial. Conversely, we should willingly accept new criteria for diagnosis and gladly adopt a more effective and safer treatment.

As we alluded to above, in 1990, a uniform system of examination was adopted to aid physicians in making the diagnosis of fibromyalgia. The Copenhagen Declaration, as this document was named, had been written by the American College of Rheumatology (ACR) a few years earlier. Its primary focus is directed to nine different, symmetrically located areas on each side of the body for a total of eighteen potential sites where physicians are urged to seek the so-called "tender points." Pain must exist in at least eleven of the predetermined places upon the application of a prescribed amount of pressure. There must be at least one painful spot in each quadrant of the body. In addition, other symptoms must fit the description of fibromyalgia, and all must have been present for at least three months.

Is this an artificial and almost whimsical way of separating fibromyalgics from the rest of the world's population? Of course it is. However, it serves a purpose in that each medical researcher and author understands what is meant when a colleague writes about fibromyalgia. It is assumed or stated that the author has followed these American College of Rheumatology criteria when making the diagnosis.

But what about the individual who does not sense pain when pressure is exerted on the predetermined sites? What if the examiner can palpate swelling, sometimes painless, in those or other locations? Should we ignore such findings? What allowance is made in this arbitrary system for those with higher pain thresholds? What about those who have pain in only ten sites? Do we tell them to "come back next year when you have the necessary eleven"? How on earth would one use this method on a four-year-old child? In our hands, the above ACR criteria have proven to be of little help, by reason of these questions and for other substantial reasons.

Physicians will normally take a careful history when dealing with any illness. We think they should also delve deeply into childhood to uncover the earliest symptoms of fibromyalgia, which would escape the more casual interview. We accomplish that goal by systematically inquiring about each symptom from a long checklist we have developed. This is important to us because, as you will read, our treatment protocol can reverse the illness. It's helpful for our patients to establish a timeline and a sense of how long they have really been sick. Reversal will move them back through the timeline we establish together at the time of our first encounter, so we're meticulous about taking a history. This is of much less importance to physicians whose goal is to medicate away symptoms, since they have no reason to be concerned about how long they may have been present.

We have certainly developed a better diagnostic process and a far more definitive method of examination for fibromyalgia. Unfortunately, its simplicity is not yet appreciated or adopted by the majority of my colleagues. We concentrate on the swollen, spastic, and contracted areas scattered all over the external structures of the body. With only a bit of training, fingers become like eyes that begin to perceive the underlying problem.

Forty years ago, when I began seeing patients with what seemed like a new disease, there were no American College of Rheumatology criteria to advise me, or to designate tender points arbitrarily. I began simply by using my hands on patients to see if I could determine what was causing their pain—a method not quite so novel to older physicians. We had always been taught to examine the places where someone hurt. It was not long before I realized how very many parts of muscles, tendons, and ligaments were swollen in my patients who complained they hurt all over. The lumps and spasms were readily palpable, especially so the more practiced I became. Maybe that's the simple reason I believed they weren't hypochondriacs faking symptoms. I could find tangible evidence corroborating what they were telling me.

As my work continued with these patients, and as I stumbled upon what would become my treatment protocol, this system of examination evolved into what we now call *mapping*. We designed a caricature of the body with a front and back view. Multiple small boxes at the bottom of the picture list nearly all of the most common symptoms we encounter in fibromyalgia. We print these by the thousands because we use them when we evaluate our fibromyalgic patients, something we do every visit. After listening to their histories, we tell patients, "For now you are only a silent mannequin and we will record only what we can palpate and not what you feel." We begin by palpating the jaw joints, the TMJs, and sweep over most of the body's external muscles, tendons, ligaments, and skeleton. We represent our findings of that examination by marking in lesions on the drawing. We carefully record their size, shape, and location. We also darken them according to the degree of hardness we perceive. This is not a search for sore spots. We do not include areas because they are tender, only palpable abnormalities—that is, what our hands can feel. In this way, the patient's subjective complaints are in fact validated by objective physical findings. We don't have to be concerned, as some specialists are, that patients are malingering, because we are working with something objective, something that can be measured and felt. If fancy new tests won't show an abnormality, it's our contention that we should go back to the one reliable test that does—an old-fashioned hands-on examination. It may not be politically correct in this day of computer-generated printouts, big, expensive machinery, and graphs—and it may not be what some doctors like to do—but it's reliable and it doesn't require any fancy equipment. We've found that a simple hands-on examination tells the story.

This initial map serves as our baseline and the only objective evidence of fibromyalgia it is possible to obtain. It amplifies and validates what we extract from our detailed medical history. We remap our patients at each subsequent visit while hiding our earlier maps from our view. Only upon completion of the examination do we retrieve the older sketches for comparison. This system has effectively permitted us to find the proper dosage of our medication and to confirm reversal of the disease. It has provided us with clusters of meaningful data accumulated on several thousand people these past forty-plus years. Based upon patient observations and our series of maps, we have learned most of what we have already related and what we will describe in the remainder of this book.

We have deliberately repeated our description of fibromyalgia though this material was thoroughly covered in our first book, *What Your Doctor May* Not *Tell You about Fibromyalgia.* If you are interested in more depth than this chapter provides, you can certainly refer to that book. We have reemphasized all the symptoms because it is important that our readers first understand the disease's full ramifications. As we continue, we will add more information to help clarify why we are able to use the same parameters for diagnostic purposes in children regardless of age. If the full spectrum of the disease is grasped, then the nuances of pediatric cases are easier to discern.

Chapter 2

Pediatric Fibromyalgia

It was with great relief that I discovered my daughter had fibromyalgia . . . because all my doctors were telling me that
there was nothing wrong with her and then asking, "What's
going on at school?" as if her pain was some psychological
problem. I am even more outraged now than when it happened. At least now I know how to treat her and when to go
to the doctor. I have spent too many evenings and weekends
in urgent care centers and emergency rooms, only to be told,
"There's nothing wrong with her," or, "See that scratch on her
knee, that's the cause of her stomach pain" (presumably a
swollen lymph node). It can't be said often enough: Get your
children checked out by a good mapper and treat them when
they are young, before they are old enough to say, "Oh, Mom.
I don't have FM and I am not listening."

—*Lisa W., California*

After reading Chapter 1, you are probably wondering why
we need a special chapter for pediatric fibromyalgia. If you

have the disease and you suspect it in your child, you are already aware of the distinct differences between the two of you. Even adults searching for their own diagnosis may have great difficulty in dependably describing their own symptoms to physicians. Doctors may not quite cower visibly during your recital, but they will certainly be confused by the day-to-day variations in symptoms that you describe. The young child has an even worse time of it. For one thing, children are poor historians. Before a certain age they will lack the necessary vocabulary to state their symptoms clearly. Older children may not understand that their complaints are abnormal.

We don't mean to imply here or anywhere else in this book that pediatric fibromyalgia is a yet-unheard-of diagnosis or one that we've invented. The diagnosis has been used in medical literature since the 1980s, often written as the acronym JPFS (Juvenile Primary Fibromyalgia Syndrome). It may not be common enough for every physician (especially nonspecialists) to have heard about, but awareness of the condition is rapidly growing. In November 2001 the American College of Rheumatology (ACR) sponsored a session about the condition, and many other associations will surely follow suit. This is the same ACR that many years ago created the official criteria for the diagnosis of fibromyalgia in adults, and now has addressed the problem in children. Their finding of differences between adult and pediatric fibromyalgia is not insignificant and coincides with our own findings. According to their presentation, children need have pain only in three sites on their body for a period greater than three months, in addition to five (instead of eleven) out of eighteen predetermined tender points, and three of ten minor criteria such as fatigue, anxiety, poor sleep, or IBS. As you've read, and will read again, we find the tender points an unwieldy and inaccurate method of diagnosing fibromyalgia, but this ACR statement confirms what we've found: Children do not usually have pain in as many areas as adults, and most do not have the full spectrum of symptoms.

Parents usually tell us they have visited several pediatricians and voiced concern about things that just did not seem quite right. They found that the minicomplaints of their child were simply brushed aside. They were often told that the youngster was merely mimicking parental complaints, usually those of the mother (recall that 85 percent of fibromyalgics are women). Other times the "Mommy, my head hurts," "my legs hurt," "my tummy hurts" are attributed to a desire for attention or an attempt to avoid doing an onerous task. Only a stubborn parent persists in the search for answers and an ear that will listen.

Understanding the nuances of pediatric fibromyalgia requires us to think somewhat abstractly. The illness must be viewed as a spectrum, with the least affected or youngest child offering the fewest clues. We have treated many children under the age of ten, including twelve four-year-olds. We recently examined a two-year-old because both her parents and her six-year-old sibling have fibromyalgia. She had symptoms but obviously could not relate them. I had to rely solely on her mother's observations and what my single finger could palpate overlying the muscles and sinews of her tiny body.

While many studies have been done on the demographics of fibromyalgia in adults, few have been done in children. When reviewing materials for this book we were surprised by a completely unexpected finding. We reviewed 190 charts done on the children in our practice, and we realized that the sex bias so clear in adult patients had disappeared. Our younger patients were equally affected, a nearly perfect fifty-fifty split between boys and girls, a fact we have since seen corroborated in surveys of the demographics of children seen in pediatric rheumatology clinics.

We are therefore embroiled in a mystery, one that intrigues us greatly. What could possibly happen, seemingly through the accelerated growth of postpuberty, that would so completely alter the ratio? Where do all the boy fibromyalgics go? Since female predominance remains throughout the decades of life, men don't just briefly lose their susceptibility but quite possibly retain that benefit forever. It is strange to us, and the dilemma remains unexplained.

There is no doubt that boys develop the same disease as girls. But something appears to happen during and following the hormonal surges of puberty. We are puzzling over the possible beneficial actions of testosterone, which is known to play a role in pain sensitivity. Larger bones and muscles could account for some of the discrepancy—but we have yet to understand the full story. If you are the mother of a son, or sons, we certainly know that you should not disregard their complaints because they are boys and therefore thought to be less likely to have fibromyalgia. It means we must be equally vigilant with our sons, at least until puberty.

We have not defined a clear age of onset for fibromyalgia, and several genes seem to play a part in the disease. We believe that there are at least two, and probably more, genetic culprits. We've witnessed fibromyalgia developing in children as young as two and in adults as old as seventy—and at all ages in between. This variation in age seems to suggest a multigenetic condition, and we predict more than a handful of genes will be discovered in the near future.

As we mentioned earlier, we've diagnosed just as many little boys as little girls with fibromyalgia. We also stated that this equal split widens after puberty to become 85 percent women to 15 percent men. However, that wouldn't alter the fact that affected males could carry one or more of the genes that cause fibromyalgia. Fathers can pass the disease on to their children, even if they themselves don't suffer from the ravages of the disease. Children with dually affected parents often cannot escape the illness and are generally stricken well before puberty.

> I can trace my FMS back to first grade. The teacher played a game with us all the time for all subjects. She would ask questions and the kid who answered correctly got to sit in the front seat of their row. If you missed, you went back a seat. Well, in every subject I was in the front desk—I remember so clearly knowing the answers as soon as she would ask the questions. Then about halfway through the year I remember feeling as if a shade had been pulled down over my face, as I could no longer understand her or come up with any answers—and now I was in the back of my row.
> —*Bonnie W., southern Illinois*

After age nine or ten and certainly by the early teens, a child can describe most of his or her symptoms in reasonable detail. Pains may arise from any muscle, tendon, or ligament just as in grownups. Fatigue and poor stamina are usually quite marked and obvious to parents, teachers, and child. Unfortunately, even at this age youngsters are not particularly descriptive and may not remember even recent symptoms. It will fall to the mother to recall many expressions of pain, functional aberrations, and emotional outbursts. Luckily, within a few months of onset the more observant parent, especially one who has fibromyalgia, should begin making the connection.

Older children are more perceptive and certainly more articulate. When a parent describes past complaints and the adolescent can outline the more recent ones, the tale becomes more cohesive. The story is then more easily interpreted, making the diagnosis somewhat simpler. Bear in mind, however, that teenagers may be obstreperous and refuse to admit being different from others and may steadfastly deny most symptoms. It is wise to make sure that your teenager is willing to be treated if diagnosed, and to sound him or her out for cooperation before dragging him or her to a doctor.

Adults should remain understanding and be prepared for the difficulty the doctor may have in making a diagnosis. Remember that there are no tests for fibromyalgia, and many practitioners simply do not know that fibromyalgia occurs in young children. Many doctors do not accept the idea that fibromyalgia is inherited. When parents sense the physician's confusion in trying to analyze the child's meager symptoms and lack of physical findings, it is time to speak up. It will be very helpful to mention that one or the other parent has fibromyalgia. Ask without fear: "Could this be the same trouble I have but at an earlier stage?" When the clinician is confronted by puzzling symptoms for which there is no easy answer, pointed observations about the immediate family history may prove very relevant. If both parents have the condition, or similar complaints, mention that as well. There is a rule of thumb we apply to our patients: The younger the child when he or she develops symptoms, the more likely both parents have fibromyalgia.

> The extreme times were not reflective of Andrew's behavior in general. He was normally a cheerful, cooperative child. My general description of him was that he was a pleasure to be with. There were other children at preschool to compare him with who were always unruly or disruptive. Certainly all children are occasionally that way. But with Andrew it was the incredible disparity between the good and bad times that should have been a clue for me that something was wrong.
>
> —*Holly S., Los Angeles, California*

Diagnosis in the very young is more easily made if the physician trusts observations made at home, usually by the mother. No one knows her child as well as she does. She is probably right in her conviction that something is wrong when she brings her offspring for medical attention. There is no use telling this woman that her child is normal because all children have complaints. At this point, she should politely insist that what might be expected from others is not usual for hers. She must present what few available hints she has been able to gather. Since this is all the physician will get, he or she had better listen carefully with an open mind and alter the examination to fit the situation.

To describe pediatric fibromyalgia, let's use the same format we did for the adult version outlined in the preceding chapter.

CENTRAL NERVOUS SYSTEM

> She had never slept soundly since birth, needing thirteen hours of sleep a night. On the playground she seemed to always lag behind her friends, saying she got too hot and tired to continue running. We tried more water, salty snacks, a hat. It didn't seem to make any difference.
>
> —*Beth C.*

Children, especially younger ones, have far fewer complaints than adults. A sweet, cuddly little darling may suddenly become oppressively cranky. We hear words such as "finicky," "fussy," "irritable," or "emotional" used to describe some of these almost hourly variations. Placating the child is often difficult despite the mother's attempts to rock, play, feed, tickle, or distract. This same child will also have periods of calm, and go weeks or even months without symptoms at the beginning.

Children may develop inappropriate sleep patterns: awakening or sleeping at the wrong time. They may rouse repeatedly during the night and crawl into bed with their parents seeking comfort. Sometimes, a youngster will awaken crying and resist all consoling efforts. The startled and half-asleep parent simply has to guess whether this is a medical emergency or simply a reaction to a bad dream. An older child may display fatigue by the unusual behavior of suddenly taking a nap without any urging, quite voluntarily. Do normal kids display such behavior at times? Certainly, but the astute observer should continue adding observations made one by one to the pattern to produce a comprehensive picture.

It is not normal for a youngster to break away suddenly from an activity he or she thoroughly enjoys. I was struck by this not long ago, when my nearly thirteen-year-old grandson, Nick, broke off playing with his cousins during a family gathering. He suddenly left the group and sat beside me. I saw his pallor and I asked what was wrong. "I've got a headache, Grandpa." His pain was limited but involved the entire right side of his head. I knew that his mother, my daughter Vivi, had suffered her initial symptoms of fibromyalgia at the age of eleven. I searched the area of his neck where nerves capable of producing such pain originate; that zone of the neck was distinctly affected. As I continued to examine him, I found many more of what I spend my working days seeking, the lumps and bumps of fibromyalgia. His subsequent rapid response to treatment eased our family's distress at learning that he too had been suffering from the disease.

An older child or teenager may suddenly be too tired to study or engage in even pleasurable activities. A student who was academically proficient gradually begins to suffer cyclic learning problems. Children may drop out of physical activities such as baseball or soccer, saying simply that they are "too tired." The earliest clues may come from an observant teacher who spots the erratic successes and sporadic failures that replace previously steady achievement. In the early stages of the illness, there are weeks or even months when the child demonstrates sparks of the former self. Lost work is made up and grades rise but, distressingly, again deteriorate. Parents may be told that their youngster suffers from an attention-deficit disorder even though he or she was once a high achiever and still has long periods of concentration. The array of impaired memory, poor concentration, and disturbed cognitive faculties has been precisely described by the word "fibrofog." In that limbo, the student is easily distracted and apathetic.

> It was not his aches or pains that made me realize my son had fibromyalgia. It was the simple observation that some days he could do his homework with little effort, and a few days later he could not write a sentence without many errors. On those days he was easily frustrated, tired, could not see or comprehend the errors he was making, or fix them. There was a desperate tone in his voice when I tried to elicit answers from him. This touched a chord in me and brought memories of my own childhood flooding back. I recalled days of not being able to spell words I knew very well. I remember being told to look them up in the dictionary but I could not because I did not have the vaguest idea what letters I was looking for.
>
> —*Claudia Marek, Los Angeles, California*

MUSCULOSKELETAL

Children are known for being brutally honest, and if they complain of a symptom continually, then listen. I found that my thirteen-year-old daughter, who has fibromyalgia, is not a complainer, so even though she was constantly having the pain, fatigue, and other problems associated with the illness she wouldn't always tell me. At school, teachers are required to send your child to the office if he or she is complaining of an illness, but the office is not required to call you unless they are sending your child home. So you don't always know many times that your child has a complaint.

—*Colleen G., California*

Aches and pains, common complaints in an adult, can escape parental attention in younger children for lack of verbal skills. Children often cry and require consoling before responding to the question, "Do you hurt somewhere?" The child may say, "My head hurts," but be unable to describe the exact location.

We began to understand many of our son's problems that had previously perplexed us. Ever since he was about two he would kick his legs when we would put him to bed. The weird thing about it was that it did not seem to be a part of any tantrum or fussiness. Nothing we would do or say seemed to make him stop this kicking. . . . Now, six weeks after starting guai, he has completely stopped this behavior. We just got back from our first follow-up and we found out that both of his thighs are completely clear of fibromyalgia now. So, in retrospect, we think we have a good idea of what the term restless legs means!

—*Cathy O., Bakersfield, California*

Frequent telltale symptoms are the so-called "growing pains." They are typically located in tissues adjacent to the knees and lower legs. They attack at any time—the child may be active or sound asleep. Parents are sometimes awakened by blood-curdling screams and the plaintive words, "My legs hurt." Growing does not cause pain; the term is an obvious misnomer. In the first year of life when a child triples his or her birth weight, he or she is not in pain. These symptoms usually begin about age eight or nine and may continue up to the onset of puberty. We asked 901 consecutive adult patients if they recalled having or being told they had growing pains. Thirty-five percent said yes. (As an aside, we believe that during the rapid growth of puberty, the body can use all of its biochemical and nutritive resources.) During the true growth spurt of puberty, which is hormonally mediated and occurs at a younger age in girls, pain and other symptoms frequently stop. Children become symptom-free and experience what we've christened a fibromyalgic gap. After puberty, symptoms usually resume, at least in girls.

As we mentioned in the beginning, older children, especially teenagers, may be in denial and only reluctantly admit to any problem. They prefer melding into their peer group and do not want to be different, especially due to an illness. Some typical responses to our questions are: "I'm tired because I stayed up too late." "My legs hurt but I sprained my knee in volleyball." "I've got the flu." They deny aches, pains, and emotional upheavals even in the presence of a parent who recalls all three. Occasionally, older children have treated us rudely, have lied in response to our direct and specific questions, and have been generally uncooperative. Parents sometimes delay taking teenagers to doctors knowing or fearing that they will behave this way. Of course, it's wise to make sure your offspring intends to cooperate *before* making a trip to see a doctor. If not, the encounter is liable to be unpleasant for all three. It's best if your child has a tangible complaint he or she is willing to have treated.

> My daughter is sixteen and a half and has all the signs of FMS and has since she was teeny-tiny. "Oh, Mom! All gymnasts and cheerleaders hurt all the time!" I'm going to have her mapped anyway, but I'm not going to start her on treatment until I have her cooperation.
> —*Roxanne, San Diego, California*

After children attain most of their adult height and weight, the danger of fibromyalgia, at least for girls, becomes progressively greater with each passing year. As adults they are genetically more likely to develop the illness than are boys, and they also mature sooner. When these symptoms begin in teenage girls, the seemingly unconnected complaints are unfortunately often brushed aside and blamed on emotional changes induced by their maturational hormone surges.

IRRITABLE BOWEL

> I don't think she is saying her bottom hurts because she knows mine does. She holds it much of the time and says it hurts. . . . She is frequently constipated and if it hurts her to have a bowel movement, she holds it in no matter how many laxatives we give her. She'll just scream for hours because she has to poop and is too scared. . . . Last time I went

to her pediatrician she asked if there was any sexual abuse. God, that is not the case at all. We are just a good, wholesome, religious, loving family with a health problem in an embarrassing spot!

—*Sandi, California*

There are few descriptive words for intestinal and excretory functions, and they are seldom among the first ones taught. Just as is the case with the other nuances of fibromyalgia, a child's immature verbal skills severely handicap his or her expression of gastrointestinal symptoms. As usual, it is the mother who must interpret and relate the symptoms she has observed. The youngest children are always difficult for pediatricians, who frequently feel as if they are practicing veterinary medicine because of the lack of input from their patients.

With younger children parents should be alerted by unexplained intestinal abnormalities that appear and vanish with equal abruptness. Mothers often tell us that their child had "terrible colic" as a baby. This is one part of the history that is rarely forgotten. Enduring a baby's high-decibel wail as he or she pulls up his or her legs and writhes in pain imprints a lasting image. We have no way of knowing if such colic is actually the harbinger of a future irritable bowel syndrome. Neither do we know what percentage of fibromyalgics experienced colic as babies. Since adult patients rarely bring their parents along on office visits, there is no way to extract such information!

If the child complains of abdominal pain, especially of short duration, it is safe to assume it's not "just something she ate." Food poisoning and more serious medical problems last for at least a few hours. It is a good rule to have children examined whenever strange and unexplainable symptoms arise. As in adults, vomiting rarely occurs as part of pediatric fibromyalgia, but brief and repetitive waves of nausea are common. If the physician finds nothing amiss and cannot make a specific diagnosis, do not simply dismiss what you have observed: Think fibromyalgia.

I recall my own such experiences at about age eight when I would stop playing with my friends or siblings, dash into the house, and head for a favorite couch. I would curl up into a fetal position and remain that way for about twenty minutes. The pain would vanish and I could return to my activities as though nothing had happened. This is a story I have heard echoed by many parents.

Younger children do not usually describe gas, but the evidence is frequently apparent! The audible expelling of gas or repeated whiffs of flatus annoy sufficiently to alert the entire family to the problem. Repetitive burping is usually an attempt to rid gas from the abdomen. (However, since most of it is sitting several feet away in the large intestine, belching seldom helps.)

Children may have bursts of diarrhea, and inadvertent soiling is not uncommon. The parent may be horrified by such occurrences in older children, but the devastating effect on the child's psyche is of greater concern. Following such bouts, constipation may ensue. We have seen at least one patient with bloody bowel movements. She was studied thoroughly by her physicians, who performed an extensive work-up including colonoscopies. A few areas of bowel irritation were located but none revealed sufficient erosion to account for bleeding. The symptom finally cleared as her fibromyalgia improved. Since such symptoms rarely appear, parents should not attribute vomiting or bleeding to fibromyalgia until all other possibilities have been excluded. (This is a good rule of thumb for all unusual symptoms.)

Often intestinal food allergies are suspected. The child is then subjected to extensive testing using various techniques. Skin testing is traumatic to the younger ones as multiple skin pricks are performed in a series. Antibody testing is a more sophisticated method that usually uncovers at least a few offending foods. It is our overwhelming experience that once rid of fibromyalgia, the child may often eat the suspected allergen without symptoms.

GENITOURINARY

> I have never been without vulvar pain. I can remember my
> mother putting cold cloths on my genital area, and scolding
> me for whatever it was that I was doing to irritate myself.
> —*Jane B., Clarendon, Pennsylvania*

Among the more frequent symptoms of pediatric fibromyalgia are those related to the urinary tract and especially the bladder. Infections often strike in those areas even in very young children. The urine may have an intermittently pungent and rather unpleasant odor in both boys and girls. It is often very concentrated and may have a deep yellow, brown, or even orange color.

When a child complains of any pain or burning upon urination, pediatricians will suspect a bladder infection. When a urine culture reveals infection, girls are often accused of wiping in the incorrect back-to-front direction after defecation or urination. When anyone suggests that faulty hygiene is the cause of the child's recurrent cystitis, the mother usually wilts under the accusation. She is the one who should have conducted her daughter's training. At other times the same symptoms occur, but no infection is found. When this becomes a recurrent problem everyone is puzzled. If both the bladder and the vaginal tract are repeatedly affected, confusion even may turn into a suspicion of adult or parental abuse.

> Our journey started in November when my then eight-year-old son came home from school with bladder spasms. Naturally we thought it was a bladder infection and treated it as such, but the medicine did not help. Within two days he had severe back problems and the next six months sent us on a wild goose chase to urologists, orthopedic doctors, nephrologists—all of whom did many tests. . . . Of course all of this showed nothing, but I was determined and knew the pain he was in. Of course there were doctors who came across the desk and said to me in a quiet tone that I might seek psychological testing, send him to summer camp, or ask if there might be a day-care worker that abused him. Of course this infuriated me more.
>
> —*Nancy E., Dallas, Texas*

Vaginal problems are present in about 30 percent of adult female fibromyalgics. There are similar although less frequent occurrences even in very young girls. The lips of the vagina may become reddened and irritated (vulvitis) and similarly affect tissues just beyond the opening (vestibulitis). Such symptoms cause little girls to tug at their underwear trying to pull clothing away from where it rubs or digs into involved areas.

DERMATOLOGIC

> By the time I was old enough to go to school, I had strange rashes on my hands and feet that were blistered, red, puffy, sweaty, and painful. The doctors could never figure out what they were caused by and my parents told me not to show them to other people because they might think that I was contagious and kick me out of school.
>
> —*Donna, Lomita, California*

We have already listed many types of rashes in the adult version of the disease. Mothers often describe one or more of these eruptions in their children. They may present as alternating types, changing from one occurrence to another. Fair-skinned children are more susceptible to these than darker individuals. Parents affected by fibromyalgia will sometimes recall similar rashes in their own early days or in the recurrences of adulthood. Past skin problems should be described to the child's doctor even when they are no longer present.

Hives may appear as isolated lesions or sometimes widely dispersed all over the body. Baby's eczema is often blamed on food sensitivities. The usual food suspects are rounded up to provide an explanation. When the next bout does not follow eating the same offender, the process of finding new culprits can be continuous.

Other children will have dry, scaly rashes near the nose, eyebrows, or scalp. Underneath the white scales is the reddened and irritated skin that constitutes seborrheic dermatitis. The skin burns and itches and scratching makes the eruption decidedly worse.

We are often shown tiny blisters on fingers and on other, unusual areas of the body, sometimes in small clusters. They suggest a herpes-type rash to the physician. They itch fiercely and the child may break the blisters, more content with the denuded, burning skin that replaces the itch.

Dry, lightly scaled, and isolated patches may appear almost anywhere. They do not usually itch and when they clear may leave a residual, lightly tanned zone. At times tiny red or clear bumps are felt when stroking the affected skin. They may be superimposed upon larger, dry areas or may arise in clusters. Most are found on the outside of the upper arms or on the lower legs, and may suggest eczema.

He told us, "I have one of those 'hot things.'" We finally figured out he was trying to describe a burning sensation in the muscles of his neck. Another interesting thing we found out from Nurse Claudia is that many times kids think this bothersome neck pain is from a tag on their shirt and will ask to have it cut off. Lance has been requesting this on all his shirts since he's been old enough to talk.

—*Cathy O., Bakersfield, California*

MISCELLANEOUS

Some of the seemingly unconnected symptoms of fibromyalgia can be the most telltale. I could always, for example, tell when my younger son was cycling because when I
would go in to wake him up in the morning, his eyes would
be gunky, sometimes almost glued shut. I would have to put
a warm, wet washcloth over them to dissolve the dried
crusty stuff on his eyelashes. When I would go into the
bathroom after one of the boys and they were cycling, there
was an unmistakable pungent smell from their urine, and I
always knew they would be hurting or tired that day.
                              —*Claudia Marek, Los Angeles, California*

There are symptoms that are difficult to fit into any of the
above categories. The following clues complete the puzzle that
is pediatric fibromyalgia.

The dry, burning, itching, and generally irritated eyes or
eyelids of the adult are not as apparent in children, but sometimes there will be redness of the sclera (the whites of the eyes)
that will be fairly obvious. Children may repeatedly rub their
eyes and, when this is accompanied by excessive tearing, provide clues that should attract closer parental scrutiny. More serious involvement will cause the tear glands to exude a gritty,
caked material on the inside corner of one or both eyes, especially in the morning upon awakening. When this has not had
time to harden into "sand" it may be sticky and look purulent.

Our four-year-old has almost always had sinus problems.
He always seemed to have a stuffy nose and tons of post-

nasal drip, which caused him to make a really gross sucking sound in the back of his throat almost constantly. He would get frequent sinus infections that were difficult to control and would always seem to come back within a few weeks. We thought he was getting sick all the time because he was in day care, so we took him out. We had allergy tests done but they were inconclusive. He would tell us that his eyes were "spicy."

—*Cathy O., Bakersfield, California*

The illness frequently promotes irritation of the nasal membranes. The child's nose may run with clear mucus or there may be chronic sinus congestion. Mucus may also back up into the inner ear and hearing impairment may ensue. Speech sometimes develops a nasal twang due to plugged passages and postnasal drip. Children are often observed rubbing their noses, sneezing repeatedly, and breathing through their mouths. You can be sure someone will decide all of this is due to allergies and will not consider the possibility of fibromyalgia.

Infection should be suspected when the nasal discharge becomes yellow or green. The constant mucous bath provides a wonderful culture medium for bacteria and viruses. Parents often tell stories of the multiple upper respiratory infections suffered by their children over the years. The increased susceptibility to infections also extends to the deeper tissues of the respiratory tree. Adult patients can recall their own repeated bouts of sinusitis, ear infections, bronchitis, and even pneumonia. Immune cells also seem to be affected by fibromyalgia. The assault the cells launch against various infectious agents can be ineffective, and the battle is often lost without the aid of antibiotics.

Although fever always raises suspicion of infection, we know that adults often run low-grade temperatures during the adverse cycles of fibromyalgia. In children, "low-grade" may even mean readings slightly above one hundred degrees. At such times parents will notice facial flushing and increased heat to touch. Because the child also becomes irritable, cries frequently, and cannot be pacified during such cycles, infection is logically suspected. Yet when fibromyalgia is the culprit, symptoms never localize to any particular system and the fever quite mysteriously clears without treatment. Fibromyalgia is an energy deprivation disease. When the body cannot generate energy, it shifts its metabolism to the production of heat, which in turn is responsible for these swings in body temperature.

Allergies appear to be caused by the release from the immune system of warrior cells that insinuate themselves deeply into the tissues under stress. There, they reveal their malfunction by releasing far more histamines than they sometimes should. Asthma is prevalent, though it usually recedes at puberty. Hay fever is also common and, right or wrong, is usually blamed for the chronic nasal congestion.

I remember my first meeting with Dr. St. Amand. Some of his first words were, "So tell me about your childhood." I was a bit stunned by the question at first, not realizing what my childhood had to do with my FM. He must have seen the perplexed look on my face because he went on to explain that with some patients there were signs going back to childhood. With that, he opened a floodgate of memories for me. I remember being as young as five and crying to my mom that my legs hurt, they were "jumpy" and they "wanted to grow out of my skin." My mother also had these symptoms and would say, "Oh, dear, she has inherited my bad leg aches." She never chalked it up to growing pains because she had experienced the feelings as well.

—*Penny Renee Trepp, Pasadena, California*

Most of us like precision far better than we do vagueness. By now the reader must be aware that fibromyalgia, especially in children, is a ghostlike disease. Just when you think you see it, feel it, or understand it, nothing gels. It seems wispy, an intangible tangle of subtleties that will not solidify. Nothing works well and the body functions marginally at best. This now-you-see-it-now-you-don't has thrown many patients and families into utter confusion. Don't think you are alone. Physicians have the same trouble.

Is it or isn't it fibromyalgia? Black and white is acceptable and decipherable. We all have trouble with the grays and the less perceptible shades. In the earliest stages of fibromyalgia, affected babies begin in the grayest of the zones. As soon as you are sure that something is wrong everything is fine again. Yesterday's symptoms may not be revisited for months but new ones will appear tomorrow. Passing years add deeper, contrasting shades that should catch the attention of an observant eye. The older the child, the more symptoms they carry into the doctor's examining room. The diagnosis is much easier when the blacks become blacker and the whites whiter.

Noticed a lack of energy, only wants to watch TV. Has a fear of doing things that are more daring. Difficulty riding a bike or skating. Growing pains in knees. Age seven bout with depression, one year on Paxil. At age nine he has tender shoulders with palpable lumps. Continues with sinus problems. Has had dental abscesses. Energy level extremely low. Having fibrofog. One day can add two plus two and the next can't. Not dyslexic. Having self-esteem problems. Waking up at night from pain. We do light massage and occasional Jacuzzi at night to ease the pain.

—*Kathie B., northern California*
(a list of her son's symptoms)

A good rule to remember: A young person has not had time to develop several diseases. In all likelihood, multiple symptoms and physical abnormalities will stem from only one condition. Alert parents as well as astute physicians are aware of this. It is basically the role of the parent, especially a fibromyalgic one, to detail past observations just as it is the doctor's task to connect this information with current complaints. The combined effort should lead the professional into performing the type of examination that clinches the diagnosis of fibromyalgia.

If fibromyalgia appears in your children, reveal what you have observed over the years to your doctor and describe the condition in detail. Your children may even surprise you by remembering more than you think when their own memories are jostled. Discuss the genetic origin of the illness with them as soon as feasible. If necessary, they, in turn, will be able to diagnose their own children in a timely manner. This is a gift you can give both your child and your future grandchildren. Give them a chance to get an early diagnosis and avoid the ravages you may have experienced.

At this point we will remind you of what we wrote above: Fibromyalgia is not a disease of black and white. There are many color zones in between, and children change as they grow and mature. We have not given you an easy one-two-three-bingo check sheet that will make the diagnosis simple. There is no such sheet. We warned you this was a bit of a ghost story. Your suspicions should be aroused. You should remember in vivid color the times of torment in your child's life. And, with or without the help of your own mother, grandmother, or aunt, you may hear echoes of your own youth. You hold the most powerful clue for suspecting the diagnosis in your own family. Once you place all the clues in context, you can blend the black, the white, and the gray moments into a complete picture. If your child had unusual complaints when young that are renewed in the later teens or early adulthood, you must resurrect your suspicions. If you are a parent with fibromyalgia you have a distinct advantage here. You the mother or you the father, perhaps both, have one up on your doctors: You know what it feels like to have fibromyalgia.

Somewhere in his young teens, Jason began to ask me if I had any good vitamins. I remember looking for vitamins or power drinks because he would mention this to me so often. We decided his diet was awful and he should try to eat better. Still, he didn't complain of any of the classic fibro symptoms. But little by little he began to do less and less. He would play baseball with his brother on a team. He would come home and plant himself in his chair. He was tired. Still I didn't see any pattern. He would try vitamins and we both agreed that he needed to eat right. One day he described to me how his knee felt. He said when he was playing baseball he had more energy but once he stopped to take a break he had a really hard time getting going. By age twenty-two he wasn't going to school or working. He was still a great kid, not hanging out anywhere, just not doing anything. Not talking about college, but he would read or play some video games. He still tried to play baseball but he said the morning games were torture and he was wiped out for the rest of the day. All along he did not verbalize that he was tired or that his limbs felt heavy, or that he had odd pains here and there. I had kind of tap-danced around the subject before but once I read about pediatric fibromyalgia I was very suspicious. I asked him questions and we went step by step through the past.

—*Jayne C., San Diego, California*

Chapter 3

Diagnosis and Treatment of Pediatric Fibromyalgia

The moral of my story: As a mother, if you suspect any of your children have FM, do something about it. I spent years listening to pediatricians telling me that my children's leg pains were growing pains (we are short and we don't grow that much). Others told me that my daughter's headaches were due to her being a nervous child. . . . It is such a relief to actually know what is wrong with my children, and now I can get them well. Dr. St. Amand emphasizes that "the mothers will diagnose their children." I KNOW he's right!

—*Kathy, Atlanta, Georgia*

MAKING THE DIAGNOSIS OF FIBROMYALGIA

When I was in the third grade I began suffering from chronic pain in my lower abdomen. My mother took me to the doctor, who, after reviewing all the medical tests he had prescribed, told my mother there was nothing wrong with me, it was all in my head. My mother said, "You mean she's making this up?" and he said, "Oh, no, she thinks she has pain, but she doesn't."

—*M. Sheridan*

There are no diagnostic tests to corroborate your suspicions or to confirm your homemade diagnosis of fibromyalgia in your child. Any and all laboratory tests prove equally unhelpful. You come away from visits to doctors totally confused because their examinations have provided you with no further information. Frustrated? You should be. If you feel that you are alone in trying to interpret the abstract symptoms your child has experienced over the years, we can help.

In Chapter 1 we described the routine used by most doctors for making the diagnosis of fibromyalgia. You will recall that most physicians do this by searching for a certain number of tender points. This sounds simple and clear-cut, but it is an arbitrary scheme that does not even work for certain adults, let alone for a squirming child. Counting tender points might be acceptable for diagnosing a teenager who has acquired most of the adult complaints, but it is totally useless for younger children. Little children hardly submit to any examinations, and the tickle factor inserts itself as a strong impediment. Usually, poking one's fingers into a child using the prescribed pressure will terminate the examination within the first few thrusts.

You will remember that we, on the other hand, examine most of the external body surface searching for abnormalities, those that we can feel without input from the patient. It is our technique that we refer to as mapping. On follow-up visits, we hide previous maps until we have completed the new one. We follow the same procedure on each return visit. This method readily shows us what has cleared, or is in the process of reversing. Thus we can tell what remains to be done, predict the speed of recovery, and ascertain the required dosage of medication.

We use this same mapping technique with children, and it helps us to confirm and make an early and accurate diagnosis. In fact, the information we gain from mapping is even more important in children than it is in adults. Their lack of verbal skills forces us to rely even more upon what our fingers can detect. Squirming is not a problem because we are not trying to locate tenderness: We can examine by merely feeling gently. A soft-stroking examination will suffice when one's fingers are sufficiently trained. (We sometimes resort to an old pediatric trick in the tickle-sensitive areas. We ask the child to play doctor and help us conduct the examination. He or she presses firmly atop our own examining fingers as we move them. Tickling vanishes and the child seems to relish participating in the procedure.)

We have taught this mapping procedure to many physicians and allied medical professionals. It is quickly learned and applicable even within the constraints of HMO or other insurance-dictated time limits. How much of the body can be examined in a given time will depend on the examiner and the speed he or she develops with experience. Often, mapping is delegated to someone with experienced hands, persons who have been trained to feel abnormalities. Patients may appeal to chiropractors, physiotherapists, or masseuses for serial mapping if their physician does not feel secure in this practice. A videotape demonstrating the technique of mapping was made for the Fibromyalgia Treatment Center in 1999 and is available through the website *www.fibromyalgiatreatment.com*. There is a nominal charge for this tape, but all proceeds are given directly to this nonprofit foundation for fibromyalgia research. For complete information please see the Resource section at the end of this book.

It is also helpful if the physician completes a check sheet or makes a list of your child's complaints. Irritable bowel is a common presentation, as are leg and back pains. Periods of fatigue, problems with memory and concentration, anxiety, and other symptoms should be noted along with their intensity and duration. As your child's map improves, so should his or her symptoms. You can keep a brief log of your child's bad and good days. This input, combined with your child's maps, should convince any physician of the reversal of the disease.

Special Tips on Mapping Children

Children certainly display far fewer lumps and bumps than adults. However, the left side of the neck (sternomastoid muscle), top of the shoulder (trapezius), and the areas inside the shoulder blade are affected in 96 percent of kids with fibromyalgia. About 84 percent have the same lumps on the right side as well.

A lump on the left thigh (front and outside), which is present in nearly 100 percent of adults with fibromyalgia, is only present in about 75 percent of

---

kids with fibromyalgia. When it is present, it is important that it be monitored, because, just as in adults, it disappears within one month of the child's taking the correct dosage of guaifenesin and avoiding salicylates.

TREATMENT: THE GUAIFENESIN PROTOCOL

He said, "I have a headache," as he lay down on the bed. I asked, "Where's your headache?" He pointed to his forehead, then neck, then down his body and legs. I said, "You have a headache in your whole body?" He answered, "Yes." About thirty minutes before he had asked for an ice bag for the outside of his calf muscle.

—*Cathy O., Bakersfield, California*

Critics might ask, why treat children so soon and with so little evidence? We invariably answer that parents know their children. If they suspect something is wrong and mapping confirms the presence of lesions, why wait? If one or both parents have fibromyalgia, they naturally wish to prevent their children suffering as they have. There's another issue as well. Parents who had this illness as children recall clearly how much this "invisible" cluster of symptoms caused them to suffer.

Luckily there are only small changes necessary in treating children as compared to adults. We use a single medication called guaifenesin, the most potent of all those we have used successfully over the past forty-one years. Guaifenesin is classified as an expectorant. Its primary purpose has been to liquefy mucus. It is often included in over-the-counter preparations used for colds such as cough medications. It permits patients to raise mucus more easily and, in so doing, lessens the trapping of infectious agents, pollens, or dust in the respiratory passages. It is also used in prescription strength for any condition where thick mucus might prove a problem, including allergic rhinitis (hay fever), sinusitis, bronchitis, or asthma.

Guaifenesin is without known side effects and has been used in some form for over four hundred years. This safety factor has allowed us to prescribe whatever amount is needed to reverse fibromyalgia, even in small children. It is interesting that the original form of guaifenesin was a bark extract, guaiacum (or guaicum), which was used for rheumatism (muscle pain) and other complaints, including growing pains in children. It still exists in this herbal form, but we find no reason to use it, since pure guaifenesin contains no plant residues, is pure, and has no side effects.

Guaifenesin is usually prescribed in a 600-milligram tablet, though 400-milligram and 1,200-milligram strengths are also available. It is also found in a 200- and 300-milligram form that may be sold without a prescription. Because this over-the-counter preparation is not as strong, more tablets are needed, so it is more expensive. There are also liquid formulations of 100 or 200 milligrams per teaspoon. This selection allows us to tailor dosages and preparations to fit the child's ability and willingness to swallow medication. It also makes it simple to adjust the amounts required for even the smallest individuals.

Readers may want to know the usual dosages of guaifen-

esin needed to initiate reversal. In the case of younger ch
it will be less than in the adult. We can frequently guess the required amount because that is genetically determined, like the
disease itself. Thus, if we know the necessary dosage for one or
more members of a family, we are usually correct in selecting
the same for the child. Some consideration is given to the
youngster's size, but the dosage modification is often slight. As
children grow, they will eventually require a full adult dosage,
generally the same level required by the fibromyalgic parent. In
the case of a dual inheritance, the amount will usually be no
higher than that of the higher-requirement parent. In a nearly
grown child, 300 milligrams twice daily will begin reversal for
only 20 percent. Six hundred milligrams every twelve hours
will initiate benefits for 70 percent, and 1,800 milligrams, 90
percent. Obviously, 10 percent require more.

We currently treat eight adults who require 4,800 milligrams (eight tablets) daily, and five who have reversed very
well on only a single 300-milligram dose daily. We have treated
a 315-pound college football tackle. He rapidly reversed at
300 milligrams twice per day. Another patient, a 118-pound
woman, requires 4,800 (eight tablets) per day both for reversal
and maintenance. Therefore, size and weight are not good in-
dicators of dosage requirements. The same applies to children.
We are fortunate that guaifenesin's safety permits using whatever dosage is needed to reverse fibromyalgia.

We begin the tiniest of our patients at 200 milligrams of
liquid guaifenesin twice daily. Older children who are able
to swallow tablets begin at 300 milligrams (half of the 600-
milligram form) twice daily, the same as the adult starting
dosage. Patients usually return one month after initiating treat-

ment, at which point we change the dosage if necessary. Our mapping procedure will inform us if reversal is under way. If not, we raise the amount to 600 milligrams twice per day and hold there for another thirty days. We continue raising the dosage on each subsequent visit until the mapping assures reversal.

If your child is old enough to relate symptoms, remember that when taking the proper dosage of guaifenesin symptoms will briefly get worse. Your child may be achy, or experience flulike symptoms, or be more tired than normal. Increased irritability will probably accompany the other complaints. When you have reached a dosage where your child feels worse, and/or the mapping shows improvement, that is the correct dosage. Your child need only take his or her medication and watch for good days to appear, and then multiply. Luckily for younger patients, good days occur fairly quickly, and cycles of pain and fatigue are soon fleeting. Your child will not remain worse for very long, particularly if he or she is still having good periods. That's the reason many parents want to start treatment as soon as possible.

For the most part, once you've found your child's correct dosage, no change is necessary. However, as children grow, some do need more medication. A periodic checkup by a doctor or a periodic mapping by any trained practitioner should catch the need for this adjustment early on. If your child has grown a great deal and begins to feel worse, it is a good time to make an appointment for a recheck.

When the child's symptoms have cleared, the genetic trait remains. Many children will quit taking medication in their later teens. It is often not acceptable to older teenagers or young adults to deviate from their peers. They are reluctant to accept medication, especially for a lifetime. They certainly feel invincible and may only vaguely recall how they used to feel.

If treatment is halted, symptoms will eventually return. Stopping and starting causes no ill effects. It does not matter if patients stop taking guaifenesin, since they have at least learned that there is such a disease as fibromyalgia. They will also recall some of its ramifications and learn the probability of recurrence with each cessation of treatment. It is easy to resume guaifenesin use when symptoms return and, if the patient does not wait long, reversal is rapid.

I told myself it was just growing pains. After a year and half of symptoms that came and went, of fatigue, and after another bout of chest pain, I was finally convinced . . . fibromyalgia was the cause of her problems, just as it had been mine, when I had been a child. . . . Knowing guaifenesin was safe for children to take made the decision for me. When I went on guai, Ember did, too. Our daughter has been on guai for months now, and she has had very few cycling symptoms, but she slept better in just about a week's time. By the end of several weeks she seemed less tired and began having an easier time keeping up with her first-grade classmates. . . . There have been no more complaints of foot and knee pain. There has been no recurrence of chest pressure or pain. Once or twice she complained to me that she ached all over. We commiserate over cycling, and I ask her if it is worth it. The answer is "yes." Does she really think she feels better on the guaifenesin? The answer is a definite yes. We take our ibuprofen and snuggle up with a video until it works. If I forget her guaifenesin, she reminds me. She isn't willing to go back to feeling bad. I'm so glad she won't have to go forty-nine years with fibromyalgia or take eight years to reverse. I am so grateful for the guaifenesin. (It's working for me, too.)

—*Beth C.*

In conclusion, symptoms are not easily extracted from younger patients. Parents can assist physicians to make the diagnosis by detailing suspicious complaints. When treating children, it is extremely helpful to have them mapped before initiating treatment, both to confirm the diagnosis and then to chart progress. Accurate mapping is often more essential in children than in adults because initially it may be difficult to detect worsening or improvement. Serial examinations should be done in the same manner at each subsequent doctor's visit. The physician should begin at low dosages of guaifenesin and raise the amount according to what the next map shows, until reversal is distinct. When improvement has been confirmed both the treatment and the maintenance dosage are established for that patient.

—⚜—

Chapter 4

Theory of the Cause of Fibromyalgia and Why Guaifenesin Works

I know that the medical community will discover that this theory is correct and in the meantime I hope that many parents will stumble upon and embrace this protocol. It is so important to have hope and never give up. There is a way out and we, along with many others, are living proof.

—*Nancy E., Dallas, Texas*

Treatment innovations usually evolve because someone has investigated an illness that sorely needed a solution. Ideally, the entire chemical sequence of the malfunction has been determined in the process, delineating clear-cut differences between a normal individual and an abnormal patient. When this is the case, drugs can usually be designed to correct or counteract the cause of the illness. Solutions arrived at in this traditional manner tend to be the ones medical scientists most readily accept and trust.

Occasionally, however, discoveries are made by sheer luck. Forty-one years ago, I was treating a man for gout, using probenecid, the only medication we had at the time for that disease. Probenecid was known to act on the kidneys to prevent the buildup of uric acid in the body. Much to my mortification, this patient reached into his mouth and stripped a few chunks of tartar off his teeth. Flicking them to my office floor, he asked me if probenecid could be the source of his newfound ability. Unpleasant as it was, his display had far-reaching effects: It eventually forced me to recognize that there was a nameless disease that affected many of my patients that I could no longer ignore.

I had been studying gout, a mostly inherited type of arthritis caused by a waste product of metabolism called uric acid. An English physician, Thomas Sydenham, beautifully described the disease about 350 years ago. He listed a large number of complaints, a prodrome, or set of premonitory symptoms, experienced by his patients beginning a few days before the joints would become painful. I observed several persons, mostly men, with episodic complaints that fit Sydenham's original description. What held my attention was that these patients did not subsequently succumb to the joint attacks expected to follow. Because this special group had elevated blood levels of uric acid, I decided to treat them as if they had gout and to see if I could improve their systemic symptoms.

When treating gout we expect to reproduce pain each time uric acid crystals are extracted from joints. In fact, the symptoms of clearing are often worse than those initiated by the untreated disease. So it came as no great surprise when, during treatment, this group suffered a forceful resurgence of all of their previous complaints. Over the course of this cyclic reversal, their attacks became less frequent and progressively less intense, similar to what happened when we treated the gouty, arthritic subjects. I gradually accumulated a large number of patients with this strange reaction. The absence of joint pain and swelling meant it was not gout, so I simply gave these symptoms the name of "uric acid syndrome."

Patients are usually drawn to doctors who specialize in poorly recognized conditions. The word spread that I was having success treating mislabeled neurotics and hypochondriacs who, I was convinced, suffered from a disease not yet described. I soon discovered, to my great discomfort, that only a small minority of these newcomers fit into my uric-acid-syndrome group. The distinct majority had most of the required symptoms but, unlike the others, did suffer multiple aches and pains. To complicate matters, their blood uric acid levels always tested normal.

I realized I was now dealing with an entirely different condition totally unrelated to gout. I also soon learned I could use the same medications to reverse it. In the beginning we called this new entity by the well-accepted name, rheumatism. Later we tried several different names, some descriptive of muscular aches and pains though hardly suggestive of much else. And because insurance companies demanded we name it something, they accepted our terminology. Thus began my saga of the disease now known as fibromyalgia.

Years later, with the name fibromyalgia in place, my patients and I were now at least vindicated with a named illness. By this time, I had also found a total of four effective medications that would reverse it. So we had a treatment and an illness with an official name, but left unanswered was the question of what caused the disease. I didn't have many clues to work with.

OUR THEORY OF WHAT CAUSES FIBROMYALGIA

Medical people usually skip right past the teeth when they examine the throat. The status of teeth is not one of our high priorities: We leave that to dentists. So I must confess my own ignorance concerning the significance of dental calculus, popularly known as tartar. I knew nothing much about its existence and less about its composition. My gouty, tartar-flicking patient had riveted my attention sufficiently to make me seek information from a textbook of dentistry. I found that dental plaque is initially soft but is rapidly mineralized and hardens. I also learned that it is formed from saliva, and is primarily made up of calcium and phosphate. I had observed that my new, non-uric-acid-disease patients usually had such deposits. Putting these meager facts together, it seemed logical that I was witnessing a metabolic disturbance, possibly evidenced by the buildup of dental calculus. If I was right, the problem was somehow related to one of the two component minerals, but was it calcium or phosphate?

We soon excluded calcium as the *prime* offender for many reasons that merit no discussion here. Calcium does play a formidable albeit lesser role that we will discuss later. This left us with phosphate. Much was already known about its chemistry, and we have learned a great deal more in recent years. We will consider faulty phosphate metabolism as the prime suspect in fibromyalgia until we can be shown a more likely villain.

Once we focused on phosphate, it was time to test our theory. We reasoned that phosphate accumulations were affecting areas of the body adversely. It followed that the reversing medications would have to increase phosphate excretion in the urine. This seemed fairly easy to test. We did a simple study using our first effective drug, probenecid. We partially stabilized phosphate ingestion by eliminating all dairy products for four days. Patients collected all of their urine for forty-eight hours. At the end of the second day we started the medication and collected their urine for two more days. We found that we were correct in our assumption: After these patients began medication, phosphate excretion increased by 62 percent. Calcium and oxalate (another by-product of metabolism) elimination also increased but in smaller amounts. We have since repeated this study using our newer drug, guaifenesin, and found strikingly similar results.

At this point we should mention that we wish measuring urinary phosphate excretion were of greater value. It would certainly help us to prove our position and help monitor reversal during treatment. It would also provide the kind of concrete statistics both patients and doctors love. However, it remains a worthless and unwieldy procedure for a few reasons. Dietary phosphate intake varies greatly from day to day and that is reflected by fluctuations in the urine. It is impractical to believe that patients could continue the perpetual dietary restrictions needed to stabilize that output. The larger problem is that the metabolism of daily living releases huge amounts of inorganic phosphate, adding to the amounts found in urine.

Great variations in energy production are demanded by daily activities, exercise, injuries, and stresses, each combining to induce wild swings in the urinary excretion of phosphates.

Anything retained by the kidneys must accumulate somewhere in the body. Why can't we then simply measure blood levels of phosphate? This isn't as simple as it would seem. The usual chemical tests normally measure phosphoric acid and not inorganic phosphate. This is to avoid including the large and variable amounts connected to serum proteins. There is another serious hitch. Phosphates are not permitted to rise appreciably in the blood since this would depress calcium levels. The parathyroid glands do not allow significant variations in circulating calcium. So calcium holds the course and the excess phosphate is refused exit into the urine and not permitted to remain in the bloodstream. Where can it go? The answer to this question holds the key to our theory of what causes the symptoms of fibromyalgia.

Too little credit is given the body for the delicate elegance of its biochemistry. Each cell has wonderful coping mechanisms that protect it from any excesses or shortages that might harm it. A cell can display awesome behavior when it responds to seemingly insignificant chemical alterations. Elements are brought into cells in surprisingly exact amounts and distributed into their tiny nooks and compartments with meticulous precision. This is true and well-accepted for all substances, including hydrogen, sodium, chloride, potassium, calcium, magnesium, zinc, and trace minerals. Less appreciated is the same precise care the body takes in allocating phosphate.

We require huge amounts of phosphate for multiple functions. Eighty to 90 percent of what we ingest is absorbed to meet those needs. Cell walls and other membranes liberally incorporate phosphate into various structures. However, far and beyond all other requirements, it is massively used to create the currency of energy. This substance, ATP (adenosine triphosphate), energizes most biological activities. Three phosphates are required for the formation of a single ATP molecule, so literally pounds of this energy-providing substance are metabolized daily, whether we are awake or asleep.

If our theory is correct, renal phosphate retention ultimately leads to accumulations within cells, more in some than in others. In an attempt to dilute the new entrant and to avoid malfunction, the phosphate buildup is accompanied by water, which produces tissue swelling. Inside the cells, phosphate and some chemical fellow travelers eventually make their way into the mitochondria, the power stations where ATP is produced. We strongly suspect that these industrial centers are where the problem of fibromyalgia is first expressed. Critical, partitioned zones within those tiny organelles are where the excess phosphate can seriously impede energy production. Many scientific papers exist affirming the serious lack of ATP within the affected muscle bundles in fibromyalgia.

The body always tries to preserve its most favorable electrical balance. Phosphate carries two negative electrical charges that must be counterbalanced. Calcium, with its two positive charges, usually travels in tandem with phosphate for this reason. Unfortunately this means we must contend with the retention of another element that also accumulates progressively within cells. It is this very calcium that helps wreak further havoc.

Calcium exerts an enormous influence over a multitude of

enzymes and genes. It directs the multiple assembly lines that convert our cells into tiny energy production mills. Nerves, hormones, or chemicals trigger reactions, but only because they promote rigorously timed and well-calibrated releases of calcium. These signals require assistance from within the cells to enforce the requested responses. Calcium is imported or released from intracellular stores and directed to well-defined and limited zones within the stimulated cells. It is there that a very precise action is exacted, the one demanded by the initial, external signals. Calcium is often referred to as the final messenger because of this function. In the body, too much of a good thing is not beneficial because the body demands a balance. To the contrary, in the biochemical context of the body it is highly detrimental.

Are you beginning to see the effects of our disturbed metabolism? More calcium whips the cell into a working frenzy, but the excess phosphate will not allow sufficient energy production to equal the demand. The buildup of calcium means that whatever the assigned duties of cells, they are being repeatedly told "Do it!" Initially, cells rise to the task and shove the accumulating offenders out of the clogged metabolic pathways to sites that least interfere with cellular activities. There are also times when energy can be resurrected from different tissues and dispersed from cell to cell. This is why fibromyalgics can occasionally find enough strength for a comparatively impressive surge of activity. The problem is that as energy deprivation deepens and becomes more commonplace, this rare moment must be spent performing a single, relatively trivial chore. Eventually there is a progressive deterioration as storage facilities are overwhelmed. Debris spills over into biological streams and ultimately obstructs the performance of the cell. This accelerating malfunction becomes clear to patients when their good days dwindle and vanish, and chronic fatigue sets in.

The body's priority is to keep essential tissues such as the liver, kidneys, and heart productive. Though wounded, the digestive system keeps us nourished but frequently at a great cost in symptoms. Our brains are the most active parts of our bodies, and thus the most easily depleted of energy. The expression "a no-brainer" is aptly applied to this type of limited cerebral function. Muscles are nearly as severely affected but seem better able to withstand the goading action of calcium. Tendons and ligaments are also considerably involved, along with the other systems that we have already discussed. At times, individual cell clusters within the affected structures malfunction more severely than others, making behavior and activity even more erratic. As the disease progresses, our cells withdraw into a protective mode and modify their expenditures. Energy is always scant, but enough is produced to avoid permanent damage to the body, until fibromyalgia gives way to osteoarthritis when the joints are finally affected. The body will not let us die from fibromyalgia, although the fatigue and pain may be excruciating.

Let's try to simplify the problem in these terms. Despite mounting excesses of phosphate, the kidneys continue their retentive ways. That, in turn, increases phosphate stores within cells and an oversupply of calcium enters as a buffer. The water that bathes the cell from the outside, called the interstitial fluid, has the same constituents in overabundance. Progressive accumulations that began in the renal tubules have ended up all over the body. And finally, they begin to gum up the works!

HOW GUAIFENESIN WORKS

The last five years on guai have been filled with many ups and downs, definitely not a straight line, and a feeling of tremendous hope as we watched both our children grow into very active, normal young adults. . . . I have much to be grateful for, as I know that the picture could have been very different had we not begun this treatment and believed with all our hearts that this was the way to go. I have never felt so strongly committed to anything in my life and only that blind faith got us through the worst of it. . . . It was worth it, as I know what the alternatives would have been. My children would have been robbed of the ability to attend school, make a living, have a social life, and in addition been in terrible pain for their entire lives.

—*Nancy E., Dallas, Texas*

Guaifenesin simply helps the kidneys open the floodgates in some mysterious way (as did the drugs we tried first). As phosphates pour out into the urine, the all-clear signal is given and the blood is then permitted to give up what it doesn't want. As the abnormally high blood phosphate levels decrease, a siphoning effect is exerted on the extracellular fluids. They now send their own accumulated debris back into the bloodstream. Next, the cells respond as the abnormal entering flow is arrested, and slowly they too extrude their excesses. In time, this purging reversal will return affected cells to their normal state, and tissue functions will be restored. Patients must continue taking guaifenesin to keep phosphates at bay and avoid the return of the problem. Guaifenesin is not a cure for malfunctioning genes. It is simply a treatment that provides the next best and safest solution.

The child's genetically defective chemistry will produce progressive symptoms, as one would expect from our observations of adults. The longer fibromyalgia goes untreated, the worse the child's symptoms will become until some relief is provided by the growth afforded by puberty. On the other hand, the speed of a child's recovery when treated is highly gratifying for parents, especially those who recall the time it took to reverse their own years of illness. Mom or Dad may have pushed and prodded their reluctant physician into making an earlier-than-usual diagnosis. It may also have taken some arm-twisting to get a prescription for guaifenesin. All this, one hopes, will be forgotten when the time comes for the most appreciative smiles a doctor will ever witness. There is no way to describe the faces and gratitude of parents whose children are restored to vibrant health. And often, there is that final reward, a wonderful hug from the mother!

Chapter 5

───── ✣ ─────

Meeting the Enemy—Salicylates

When telling close friends about FM, I now describe it as a metabolism problem on the cellular level that has caused a buildup of phosphates in the body that does not allow muscles to relax. The guai allows our kidneys to excrete it. Salicylates prevent the kidneys from doing this. No one has asked to know more, and it gets the main points across. Just a few salicylate examples, like no mint toothpaste or gum. Also, with kids, you can gradually address the salicylate issues, a few at a time, over time, so they don't freak.

—*Christie P.*

There's a wise saying that if something seems too good to be true, it probably is. And unfortunately, guaifenesin is no exception to this rule. We've introduced you to a medication with no side effects that is generally effective in nice, low doses. You don't have to worry about drug interactions with other medications when you take guaifenesin—it is not contraindicated for use with any other compound. While it's true that it doesn't make fibromyalgia go away instantly, once it has cleared your symptoms, if you keep taking it, it will keep them away for life. So what's the catch?

Guaifenesin has only one enemy, a chemical foe that completely blocks its effectiveness. This is a compound known as *salicylate,* first discovered in plants. It is now known that *all* plants produce it as a protective agent against bacteria. Without salicylates or salicyclic acid, plants would never get out of the ground alive. Natural salicylates have been used medicinally for at least two thousand years, originally in the form of teas made from barks, leaves, and meadow grasses. Peoples as diverse as the American Indians, Europeans, and the Chinese knew of the medicinal benefits of salicylates for treating pain. Originally, all salicylates were extracted from plants—the name is derived from the Latin word for the willow family, *salix.* Today, salicylates are easily manufactured in laboratories so there are both natural and synthetic compounds. The best known and most commonly used is a graybeard of drugs, good old aspirin, acetyl salicylic acid, first produced synthetically in 1893.

Aspirin has been well studied from every possible angle, and we certainly know many of its effects on the body. It is our most inexpensive analgesic. It is especially effective for arthritis, musculoskeletal pain, and headaches. It works by reducing inflammation and will bring down a fever. The drug diminishes the risk of strokes and is effective in reducing damage from heart attacks if it's chewed during or immediately afterward. It may prevent certain types of cataracts and afford protection against some colon and rectal cancers. Salicylic acid is also used topically; its name appears on the label of many skin products. Its acidic nature endows it with antifungal properties, useful in products such as wart and corn removers, dandruff shampoos, sunscreens, acne medications, and mouth-washes.

Salicylates are also present in food plants, with especially high levels found in berries, some nuts, vegetables, and fruits. They are added almost surreptitiously to certain products both as flavorings and as preservatives. Luckily, for our purposes, we do not need to be concerned with the salicylates in foods, but they are present, and it has been underscored in medical liter-ature that consumption has risen dramatically in the past decade. Since salicylates are easily measured in the blood and urine, studies have been done on the changing levels resulting from various diets. It is clear from these studies that foods add insignificant amounts to the urine and to the bloodstream. Thus far, no ill effects have been documented from the in-creased ingestion, a finding that confirms our own experience that salicylate-containing foods do not enter into the guaifen-esin equation. *We cannot repeat too often, no diet is required for fibromyalgia.*

So how do salicylates create a problem for guaifenesin? The answer is quite simple. Guaifenesin, and our other successful medications, need to have access to receptors in an area of the kidney known as the renal tubules. All cells have thousands of receptors, each receptor acting like a tiny stall in a parking garage. Each is precision-made to have a unique affinity for specific messengers. For any substance to induce a desired ef-fect on the body, it must first find a properly fitted niche in a receptor. This applies to hormones, the body's natural messen-gers, as well as externally or internally generated chemicals.

The science of pharmacology relies greatly on this natural proclivity.

Medications are designed to snuggle into various receptors and thereby trigger or block a stimulating effect. Unfortunately, salicylate better suits the renal tubule receptors and very little is needed to occupy the all-too-few available sites. Because "parking spaces" are sparse, guaifenesin can be easily turned away by the competition. Such rejection means zero help for fibromyalgia. Increasing the intake of the drug will not improve the traffic snarl. In a nutshell, in the presence of salicylates, guaifenesin still loosens mucus but has no effect on the kidneys. In the real world of reversing fibromyalgia, there is no way out but to avoid salicylates.

You'll undoubtedly come across physicians and pharmacists who will try to tell you that salicylates are not as much of a problem as we have found them to be. We vehemently disagree with this poorly informed opinion. Years of experience have given us huge amounts of documentation to confirm what we say. Too many patients' body maps have illustrated the complete reversal of previous improvement when salicylates were added. Sensitivity to blockade is genetically determined and we have seen some patients blocked even by small amounts. As none of us knows our personal susceptibility, we should meticulously abide by the protocol. Give guaifenesin a fair chance. What we have written here we have learned the hard way, and at the expense of someone's hard-fought progress. Trust us when we plant our feet and say that our stance has already been tested too many times, and been proven right!

We repeat ourselves to stress the point. Because guaifenesin and salicylates blend without any adverse drug interaction, patients have no way to tell when guaifenesin's renal effects are totally blocked. Mix them accidentally and you won't know you've done it. Do it consistently, and you'll suddenly realize it when you do not improve or lose the precious ground you've gained. Since you have no short-term way of recognizing the blockade you must simply know what salicylates are and meticulously avoid them.

Remember the old "animal, vegetable, or mineral" game? You and your children can play this game to avoid plant derivatives. Anything that's animal or mineral won't block guaifenesin. Any time you or your child spot plant names on any medication, vitamin, or topical product, you need to take a closer look at the product. Cucumber, rose, mint, and aloe are words easily identified by all but the youngest. Other names ending with -root, -leaf, or -bark provide easy enough clues to suspect a problem. Less commonly known names such as arnica, jojoba, and yucca may require the use of a dictionary. Occasionally, a book on herbs is needed for precise identification.

One plant-extracted compound poses a hidden problem so you must memorize the name. Its name is *bioflavonoid,* and there are several varieties, some containing heavy amounts of salicylate. Luckily, it is usually listed and only added to supplements, most often vitamin C.

Because of the danger of Reye's syndrome, most parents know they should shun aspirin in younger children. Acetaminophen (Tylenol, for example) is preferred for use in children, and it won't block guaifenesin. Neither will ibuprofen (Advil or Motrin, for example) or any of the other nonsteroidal anti-inflammatories. It is slightly more difficult, however, to avoid salicylate when it's part of a chemical name such as ethyl or octylsalicylate (found in many sunscreens), bismuth subsalicylate (found in Pepto-Bismol), or methyl salicylate, which is found in products like Listerine and Ben Gay. Even so, the chemical name salicylate is clearly visible in those names, and can be spotted with only a little practice. In January 2002 the FDA changed the ingredient octylsalicylate to octisalate, which is slightly different, so be sure to watch for this variation too.

Intake of natural salicylates is on the upswing, especially in the form of herbal medications used even on children. Plant medications are still medications—many sufficiently potent to have far-ranging effects on our bodies. Many of these effects are still unknown, and new ones are being discovered yearly. Unlike the foods we eat, these herbal compounds are concentrated, making them powerful enough to override the liver's detoxifying capacity. If they were not, they wouldn't work as medicines. You can't make a headache go away by eating two almonds, though almonds contain a fair amount of salicylate. Even foods with greater salicylate content, such as berries, fruits, vegetables, herbs, and spices do not block guaifenesin, since the liver is equal to their challenge. We repeat because of numerous past misinterpretations: *No dietary changes need to be made when you use guaifenesin.*

Since this book is focused on children, we should stress one more thing before leaving the subject of natural salicylates. It is no secret that the Food and Drug Administration (FDA) sets no standards for dietary supplements and herbal medications. That unfortunately guarantees that the quality of those products varies greatly depending on the manufacturer's integrity. Herbs are often imported from Third World countries where they may have been grown and harvested in question-able surroundings or treated with unknown chemicals. In an era of mounting concern about pesticide residue, hormone ad-ditives, and fertilizers, the popularity of these natural remedies is somewhat ironic. There have also been numerous news re-ports and journal articles exposing natural remedies that have been laced with prescription drugs in an attempt to boost the efficacy of the natural plant. Be sure to check all vitamins and supplements for herbal additives. Be sure vitamin C doesn't contain rose hips, for example. Check the labels for names like horse tail, ginger, or licorice root. There are plenty of "plain" vitamins with only vitamins and minerals on the label.

Natural does not mean safe, pure, or nontoxic. A child who ingests certain plants from our gardens can be in as much danger as one who swallows medicine out of the bathroom cabinet.

Pure chemicals extracted from plants, other than salicylate itself, will not block guaifenesin. The process of extraction and purification is accomplished in such a manner as to insure the elimination of all other plant residues. Purified enzymes, fats, or chemicals isolated from plant sources are acceptable for use with guaifenesin. In this category are compounds such as al-phahydroxy acids, stearic acid, citric acid, beta-carotene, shea and cocoa butter, coconut fatty acids, starches, proteins, glyc-erides, waxes, gums, and so on.

Some other plant products may be used with guaifenesin. Specifically, soybeans do not contain salicylates, nor do grains such as corn, wheat, rice, or rye. They are found in other seg-ments of their plants, however, such as the leaves, roots, and stems. For example, wheat and barley grasses should not be used in any significant concentration. A more extensive list of ingredients that should and should not be used is posted at the guai-support group on the Internet at *www.netromall.com/ guai-support*. A list of products that can be used is also posted there, and on the website *www.fibromyalgiatreatment.com*. Our final word of admonition is this: When in doubt, don't use it. *Don't risk it,* don't use it. Restoration of your health is more important than any other thing.

> The skin was believed to be a nearly perfect barrier that prevented chemicals applied to it from penetrating the body. This belief went unchallenged until the 1960s when the much-heralded but unmarketed DMSO proved its ability to carry substances with it through the skin and into the body's tissues and bloodstream. . . . It has now been accepted that all chemicals penetrate the skin to some extent and many do it in significant amounts. What degree of absorption is there when a cosmetic is left on the face (as a makeup base might be) for twelve hours or spread all over the entire body (as a suntan lotion may be)? . . . Most consumers and cosmetic companies are concerned with allergic reactions and skin irritations, but what of systemic absorption, toxicity and chronic effects?
>
> —Ruth Winter, *The Concise Encyclopedia of Cosmetic Ingredients*

In the above paragraphs we've repeatedly mentioned the presence of salicylates in topical products such as sunscreens, mouthwashes, and creams that are used for muscle pain, without any elaboration. So now it's time to explain this problem in more detail because it's very important. The skin is our largest organ, and it is of course highly visible. Children burn it, bruise it, scrape it, and cut it, often on a daily basis, and teenage girls, like adult women, seek to improve and beautify it.

The skin absorbs many chemicals—witness the increase in prescription medications approved by the FDA for transdermal use. Drugs are put into skin patches and also added to chewing gums, nasal sprays, and suppositories. The main benefit of such delivery is that it permits the use of smaller dosages by avoiding destructive digestive juices. Side effects such as gastric irritation can be avoided as well. By this direct method, compounds are also able to avoid alteration by the liver. After passing through the skin, they are widely dispersed by the bloodstream.

Unfortunately for us, salicylates are one of these compounds that are readily absorbed through the skin, which poses no barrier to its entry and widespread distribution. This is obvious because were it not so, products such as Aspergum, Aspercreme, and Ben Gay would be useless. In addition, there are many excellent scientific studies documenting increased blood levels of salicylate following topical application of these and many other products. Once into the bloodstream, considerable quantities bypass detoxification by the liver and are directed to the kidney renal tubule receptors—exactly where we want no salicylate interference. Remember our analogy? Once garage spaces are occupied by salicylates, guaifenesin will find no parking, and our protocol is doomed to failure.

Salicylates are highly concentrated in oils, gels, and other plant extracts. It takes many pounds of leaves to make mint or rosemary oils and aloe gel, pounds of cucumber to make cucumber extract, castor beans to make castor oil, and so on. This concentration process guarantees that each drop of oil, gel, or extract contains more salicylates than we would ever consume by eating the lesser amounts in our food. This is why there is no problem with touching or eating any food. Obviously, holding or swallowing a handful of almonds is different from rubbing almond oil into the skin.

Salicylates are commonly found in topical products applied on children. They are found in sunscreens (aloe, octyl-salicylate, or octisalate), bubble baths, some baby lotions and powders, and in products such as baby wipes. Shampoos and conditioners should be checked for plant oils or bark extracts and other salicylates. Most medicated rubs such as Vicks contain plant oils and must be avoided. Baby lotions are primarily mineral oil, though some contain aloe and should be replaced with brands that don't. Be sure to check bubble baths, bath oils, and soaps, especially the liquid ones. Each and every product you apply to your child's skin will need to be examined. The younger the child, the fewer products you will normally need. This somewhat simplifies your task.

Toothpastes pose a special challenge because their manufacturers are not legally required to list all their ingredients. Large brands such as Colgate add mint, even to their fruit flavors. It is better to be safe and use Tom's of Maine's strawberry or orange-mango flavors or the toothpastes offered by Grace Dental Products or Andrea Rose. These can be found in the Resources section of this book.

Older children use many products such as lip balms that might contain castor oil, aloe, camphor, or menthol (mentholatum). Deodorants may contain castor oil as well. Shaving creams and after-shave lotions should be checked for ingredients such as aloe, witch hazel, or menthol. Baby oil, lanolin, and vitamin E are safe. Razors produce microscopic cuts as they abrade the face and legs. Therefore, avoid those with aloe strips. Acne medication and dandruff shampoos can pose a strong salicylate challenge, but there are alternatives.

We've warned our adult patients about gardening barehanded. Most children may pick a flower or two, or help to rake leaves, but won't be doing the kind of labor that gets plant juices and saps all over the skin. However, if your child does want to help you with this kind of work, be sure that he or she wears canvas or rubber gloves just as Mom and Dad must.

You may not have given it much thought, but medications can be absorbed through oral membranes. Both synthetic (artificial) and natural mint oil are potent salicylates and must not be used. Do not allow the use of mouthwashes, toothpastes, breath savers, or gum from any members of that family, including spearmint, peppermint, and wintergreen. Fruit, bubble gum, and cinnamon flavors pose no threat. Lozenges that contain eucalyptus, mint, or clove oil will need to be avoided as well.

As we stated above, synthetic salicylates are the easiest to spot because the word salicylate, or salicylic acid, appears on the label. Aspirin may be listed on labels as ASA (a common designation for acetylsalicylic acid), although this is more commonly done in Canada and Britain than in the United States. Children who are learning to read may think it is fun to help you look for the letters that start the word that they must learn to avoid.

Synthetic salicylates can also be found in mouthwashes, where they are listed as salicylic acid or methyl salicylate. Also be sure to avoid menthol and camphor, which are mint derivatives. Lotions and soaps used for acne, dandruff shampoos, and wart removal products may also harbor the offender. Some names, such as Sal-Clens Shampoo, Salonpas patches, or Hydrisalic are dead giveaways, but other names such as Clear Away or Freezone provide no such clues. Labels are there to rescue you from mistakes—read them!

> Kids must buy into the protocol with all it entails, or it can be very frustrating for those who are trying to help them. I am fortunate that three out of four are willing to do what it takes to get and stay well. I do believe that sometimes it takes suffering to engage people or do what it takes to get and stay well. It is especially difficult for boys to admit not only to themselves but to others that they have a problem (a macho thing!). But once they feel better that becomes the motivation . . . for all of us.
>
> —*Lori R., Irvine, California*

SALICYLATES AND COSMETICS (FOR TEEN ANGELS AND THEIR MOMS)

My goal has always been to tell you everything the cosmetic companies won't tell you and everything that the fashion magazines leave out or can't tell you because of the control that cosmetic companies assert via their advertising dollars. There's a lot to tell. Some of it you may find shocking, funny, enlightening, and depending on how much money you've wasted, disheartening.

—Paula Begoun, *Don't Go to the Cosmetics Counter Without Me*

Many adult women taking guaifenesin lament the loss of their cosmetics, and some have been known to give up the protocol to use their favorite lipstick. If grownups feel that way despite years of suffering from pain and illness, imagine the struggle that lies ahead of you if your daughter has fibromyalgia. Teenage girls want to use the latest products, the ones their friends use, or those they see in provocative magazine ads that promise dramatic results and irresistible beauty.

The restrictions we must impose provide you with a singular chance to help your daughter understand the cosmetic industry. It will be an education that will serve her well in the long run. All women should learn that companies have no obligation to prove their claims. A careful scrutiny of advertising hyperbole reveals disclaimers such as "the appearance of," "the look of," and "in some cases." No one regulates claims made on cosmetic labels.

The fact that the cosmetic companies are suddenly shoveling plant materials into ordinary moisturizers and makeup is only a marketing tool. Very few such extracts have been shown to have any appreciable benefit to the skin. Strong, irritating chemicals must be added to cosmetics with botanical ingredients merely to preserve the freshness of such things as cucumber extract. More than a few of our patients have been astonished when they stopped using so many compounds and were promptly rewarded by skin improvement.

The issue of natural versus synthetic is one that I've written about extensively over the years. To sum it up succinctly, natural does not mean good and synthetic does not mean bad. . . . I would no sooner accept any plant as being good for my skin than I would walk naked through a patch of poison ivy assuming because it's a plant it must be OK. "Natural" simply defines the source of the ingredient; it tells you nothing about the ingredient's effectiveness or risks. Menthol and peppermint may have a natural source but both are serious skin irritants and are absolutely terrible for the skin. Ingredients like silicone and stearyl alcohol are synthetic but they are remarkably silky-soft ingredients vital to a vast array of cosmetic formulations.

—Paula Begoun, *Don't Go to the
Cosmetics Counter Without Me*

If you and your daughter haven't discovered Paula Begoun's *Don't Go to the Cosmetics Counter Without Me*, you must. The author also publishes a newsletter and has a website. She reviews thousands of products, from Almay, Avon, and Cover Girl, to Lancôme, Dior, and Charles of the Ritz, with astonishing findings. She underscores that results are what matter; price and exotic ingredients do not guarantee a better product. Readers are given an inside look at the way cosmetics are conceived, manufactured, and marketed. Gaining insight is important and especially helpful to young girls who are the new targets of advertising. Ms. Begoun offers tips on caring for various skin types, acne, and how to avoid sun damage and acne. If you are daring enough to preach to your daughter about the beauty industry, Ms. Begoun can help you.

Although it certainly seems complicated at first, checking cosmetic labels soon becomes routine. Lip glosses and balms made with castor oil cannot be used, but many are made with lanolin or mineral oils. Mascaras that do not touch the skin are no problem, just as nail polishes cannot block guaifenesin. Hair conditioners containing natural balsam or plant oils must be replaced by products free of these ingredients. Recent scientific evidence suggests that sunscreens made from avobenzone, titanium dioxide, and zinc oxide are far more effective than those with salicylate formulas. Toners with witch hazel must be discarded in favor of acceptable preparations. Acne products containing salicylic acid are often too irritating for some skin types. There is a wide selection of equally effective, safe products made with triclosan or benzoyl peroxide.

It is absolutely possible to find good, high-quality products in all price ranges and for all skin types while totally avoiding salicylates. Thousands of women, armed with dictionaries and the desire to get well, have proven this repeatedly at cosmetic counters all over the world. You can help your daughter to join their ranks.

Children can participate in screening products for salicylates almost from the beginning. Gradually, as they grow older, they will become more involved in the process, but even the little ones can be told that they have to avoid such plants as mint so their medicine will work. In time this avoidance will become second nature to them, and of little consequence. Screening products for salicylates is hardly a monumental task. It is one of the least difficult tasks that children face as teenagers, and later, when they strike out on their own.

Adherence to the advice in this chapter will determine

your child's success. It sounds harsh, but it's almost that simple. Our greatest source of treatment failure is simply careless checking of labels, usually as a patient starts to feel better. As it is true in adults, so it is with children. Our reward and theirs can be accomplished only by working together to enforce what is written here.

Chapter 6

Hypoglycemia, Carbohydrate Intolerance, and Fibroglycemia

During our first appointment, Dr. St. Amand asked us if we noticed any unusual behavior if our son eats sugar. When we told him we had to cut out sugar from Lance's diet, he asked us, "Does he become belligerent?" He knew exactly what we were talking about. He told us that belligerence is what hypoglycemia does to a child. Now, at four years old our son is learning what high carbohydrate intake does to him. We recently cheated on the diet because we were out of town. After eating corn chips, beans, rice, and tortillas, we practically had to peel him off the ceiling. Needless to say, we are so grateful for the diet.

—*Cathy O., Bakersfield, California*

Although based firmly in science, medicine deals in nuances and educated guesses, which is why it is often referred to as an art. Most illnesses do not present in black and white—two extremes with no shades in between. To the contrary, there is a spectrum of possibilities, and diseases reveal themselves accordingly. Patients come in different colors, heights, and weights, each with a different personality and ingrained personal habits. Their unique genetic construction is responsible for the metabolic variations that sometimes confound us.

Fibromyalgia is composed of so many symptoms that it shouldn't surprise us when it affects one person quite differently from another. So many systems are affected by the altered chemistry that their interplay easily befuddles both patient and physician. The disease presents with a series of seemingly unconnected complaints. An overwhelming symptom may improve tomorrow only to be replaced by what today is merely an annoyance.

But on a deeper level, all of the complaints of fibromyalgia are interwoven and are easily reduced to a single common denominator. We have discussed the ubiquitous energy deprivation that has an enormous effect on central nervous system function. The brain has an overriding instinct to take care of itself. That behavior is sometimes beneficial, but occasionally signals are misinterpreted and the brain acts detrimentally. Foods are fuels and energy production requires fuel. The brain's selections are often driven by its innate perception of only its short-term and immediate metabolic requirements.

Fibromyalgics are tired all over. In the past, eating effectively altered this situation by stoking the physiological furnaces that produce energy. The preferred quick fix for energy is carbohydrate (sugar or starch) because it raises blood glucose within a few minutes of ingestion. Therefore, as they get sicker, fibromyalgics begin craving carbohydrates as the body vainly tries to make more energy. Often they yield to overpowering carbohydrate cravings and devour candy bars or potato chips. However, as we will see, succumbing to that urge may create serious metabolic consequences and actually create further energy deprivation.

> There are other things . . . such as having night terrors. Very alarming for the parent. Supposedly of no consequence to the child, but I never want to go through those again. Andrew had them from the time he was maybe eighteen months until he was perhaps three. He may have had a few since then but the crying was not the hysterical screaming of the earlier ones.
>
> —*Holly, Los Angeles, California*

Hypoglycemia (low blood sugar) is traditionally defined as a blood sugar level below fifty milligrams per deciliter. The standard five-hour glucose tolerance test used to diagnose blood sugar problems is performed after the ingestion of a heavy carbohydrate load. It will, however, miss many, even severely affected, patients because samples taken at preordained intervals may simply miss the blood sugar's nadir, or lowest point. Recent reports have corroborated another equally important fact. Full-blown symptoms occurred in healthy young people at what are considered perfectly normal blood sugar readings. We must therefore diagnose hypoglycemia from its symptoms and not on the basis of blood tests.

To better understand hypoglycemia and the symptoms we use for diagnosis, we need to take a closer look at what happens when we eat carbohydrates. All carbohydrates, foods such as sweets, bread, pasta, rice, and potatoes, cause the blood sugar to rise rapidly, which stimulates the pancreas into releasing insulin. This rapid response begins well before we finish eating. Insulin is responsible for driving glucose into cells to serve immediate or future energy demands. Its effectiveness as a storage hormone allowed the human race to survive periods of famine and scarcity.

As glucose is taken out of the blood to be used or stored, blood sugar levels return to normal. But certain people are unable to process carbohydrate loads properly. Hypoglycemia ensues when there is an excessive release of insulin or a delayed or inadequate release of the other hormones that are supposed to stop the rapidly tumbling blood sugar.

The brain has receptors for glucose, its basic fuel. When the blood sugar falls too low, it senses deprivation and decides it must protect itself from death at the price of some uncomfortable consequences. In its panic it fires a salvo of its most potent weapons, the so-called counter-regulatory hormones. First, growth hormone is launched from the arsenal, but it unfortunately requires four hours to effect a rise in blood sugar. Next, the brain orders the adrenal glands to release cortisol, but four hours will elapse before it can provide significant relief. As the blood sugar continues to fall, the brain enlists another ally, and the pancreatic hormone glucagon dutifully responds. Even it will require about twenty minutes before it can make an effective assault.

If this much time were to elapse, the insulin attack would prevail. Blood sugar would continue a perilous free fall and the ensuing hypoglycemia would seriously imperil survival. Luckily, the brain has a combat ace at its disposal: adrenaline from the adrenal gland. Unfortunately, this fail-safe hormone delivers relief at a considerable price!

We have all experienced adrenaline rushes. Epinephrine, its medical name, is the "fight or flight" hormone that is immediately released when we are startled. Such surges are evoked by a threatened assault, a suspected intruder in the home, or by hearing horrible news. The body warns of impending disaster with heart pounding, hand tremor, clammy sweat, frontal-pressure headache, and great anxiety. Internally induced alarms produce the same sensations. As we have seen, significant falls in blood sugar deeply frighten the brain and produce the identical reaction. When adrenaline release causes these symptoms unexpectedly during the night it is usually attributed to nightmares. By day, it is likely labeled a panic attack.

Most hypoglycemics suffer repeated adrenaline assaults that cause the acute symptoms we have just described. But, like adults, older children manifest many chronic complaints that are also part of the hypoglycemia syndrome. The metabolic disturbances result in fatigue, irritability, nervousness, depression, insomnia (usually frequent awakening), impaired memory and concentration, anxieties, sugar craving, dizziness, and occasional fainting. In fact, it is not uncommon for the irritable bowel syndrome to appear as part of these chronic symptoms. Therefore such things as nausea, gas, bloating, constipation, and alternating diarrhea should be added to the chronic panoply of complaints. Are you beginning to visualize the amazing symptom overlap of hypoglycemia and fibromyalgia?

Unlike adults and older children, younger children do not

display the usual symptoms we have just listed. Their adrenaline spurts trigger a different scenario. Most gently stated, they demonstrate very irritating behavior. They are moody, burst into tears without provocation, throw temper tantrums, become aggressive and hyperactive. These are their equivalent acute symptoms. The observant parent will also observe hints of the chronic symptoms. Younger children may wander around the preschool room, ignore others at play, and take unsolicited naps. They may scream in the night and parents will suspect a nightmare. Are they also depressed, confused, anxious, and frightened? How will they tell us?

Mothers soon figure out that feeding helps their cranky children. Carbohydrates such as candy bars, sugared drinks, starches—anything that quickly raises blood sugar—will render them docile within as few as five minutes. However, this unfortunately only perpetuates the problem by inducing yet another insulin surge that will induce identical symptoms two to four hours later.

Almost seven years ago, a study was published relating to diet and hyperactivity. Two groups of children were tested. One was composed of elementary school children whose parents had identified them as adversely responsive to sugar. A similar number of purportedly normal children composed the second group. Sucrose (table sugar) was liberally included in one diet, but considerably restricted in the other. Each diet contained approximately equal calories. The usual complex carbohydrates, including potatoes, pasta, and rice, were not removed. Diets were switched at appropriate times in this blinded study; neither parents nor subjects knew whether sucrose or aspartame was used as a sweetener.

No differences in behavior were noted in the parent-described sugar-intolerant children on both diets. The children continued their hyperactive, belligerent ways. Since their abnormal behavior prevailed at the same frequency with both sugar and aspartame, the authors concluded that sugar consumption was not a factor in hyperactivity.

Physicians readily accepted these unexpected results since they were published in a very prestigious journal. However, it was no surprise to us that both groups continued to be irascible little hellions. This journal declined to print our letter that pointed out a serious flaw in the study. We reminded the editors that potatoes, pasta, and other complex carbohydrates are rapidly converted to glucose within the body, only a bit more slowly than sugar. For example, potato starch is merely a string of glucose molecules. It starts converting to glucose within two minutes, even as it is being chewed. Our rebuttal stated the obvious: This elegant study was worthless. With their dietary substitutions, the researchers had simply compared the effects of sugar to those of sugar!

> Once I began to really question him I found that he suffers from fibrofog almost as bad as I do. He described reading a chapter and by the time he got to the second chapter he forgot where he was or what the chapter was about. But on his own he had never complained about this. I think he, like me, thought everyone else felt like this. We took him to Dr. St. Amand and he does have fibro, his map was pretty full. I think it was a relief to my son to realize that he had been sick and not incompetent.
>
> —*Jayne C., San Diego, California*

We have seen many older children who have been diagnosed with attention deficit disorder. Yet, many of them functioned very well at one time, and may still do so in spurts. Parents tell us that their previously excellent grades are now either attained with great difficulty or have rapidly fallen into mediocrity. Many have dropped out of school and have been relegated to home tutoring by despairing parents who seek to reverse their academic decline. Younger children may seem somewhat dazed at times, suggesting the same problem. They seem to learn only with difficulty, which is often blamed on inattention. Some children or teenagers are tortured by labels such as ADD, ADHD, or learning disabled, which cause reverberations throughout their school years. They may remain stigmatized well into adulthood.

FIBROGLYCEMIA

Early on I abandoned the idea of birthday parties for Malcolm. The sugary treats, the cake and ice cream created a monster an hour or two after he ate them. And, since it was his party, the tantrums he threw were particularly hard to deal with. I could not scoop him up or take him home, he was the host. He would be stubborn, cranky, selfish, and intractable. He was downright unreasonable, and would go into a full-blown tantrum when he was crossed. I knew it was the effect of the sugar, like a drug taking hold of him. When his fibromyalgia was bothering him and he was cycling, his blood sugar swings were worse, and more frequent.

—*Claudia Marek, Los Angeles, California*

The brain requires more energy ounce for ounce than any other bodily structure. When fuel-deprived and hypoglycemic, it is hardly able to download new data into its memory bank. A child or adolescent cannot be attentive if deprived of well-functioning energy generators. Ask any fibromyalgic adult how well his or her concentration and memory centers function. They will describe fibrofog in detail and allow you to grasp how our children react as they sink deeper into this same morass. Plug hypoglycemia into the equation and perhaps add even a modicum of actual attention deficit disorder. Drag these children to some unsuspecting physician, relay all the information that the child cannot articulate or sits there denying, and try to get a diagnosis.

Fibroglycemia is a name we coined in our first book to describe the overwhelming combination of fibromyalgia and hypoglycemia. The two conditions intertwine into a duo that produces some of our most chronically ill adults and children. Individual cells of fibromyalgia as well as the contracted muscles, tendons, and ligaments labor mightily, expending fuel day and night. Their system-wide, twenty-four-hour-a-day overwork creates a huge demand for energy.

Forty percent of our female fibromyalgics suffer from carbohydrate intolerance or hypoglycemia. This increases the chances their daughters will follow the female pattern. Sons are less likely to succumb and only about 20 percent become carbohydrate-intolerant, as is the case for adult males. During our many years of treating combined fibromyalgia and hypoglycemia in adults and children, we have found no shortcuts. We must attack fibroglycemia on both fronts. We ask our parents to follow the prescribed diet that corrects hypoglycemia and at the same time we institute treatment for fibromyalgia with guaifenesin.

We follow the same protocol with younger children who present with fibromyalgia and hyperactivity. Aware that we will not see the usual adult presentation, we accept the mother's description of aberrant behavior both in school and at home. It is sufficient diagnostic evidence. Who else should we trust? The mother's observations make hypoglycemia likely, and our mapping confirms fibromyalgia.

Just as for adults, there is no point in delaying the treatment of fibromyalgia while awaiting the dietary reversal of hypoglycemia. We urge the mother to enforce the diet as best she can as we begin guaifenesin. We choose whatever form will best suit the child's age and ability to swallow. Our gratification comes quickly with children. Their response is swift, and our little bandits quickly convert to delightful companions.

Adults begin to respond to the proper diet within four or five days, and are 75 percent better in one month and totally clear after two months. Children can seem outwardly improved within the first day. Behavior changes both at home and at school are usually quite visible within a week or two. After careful adherence to the diet for one month, they can be allowed some judicious cheating, just as we adults are permitted after two.

It should be anticipated that each child will resolve the problem differently. Please remember how we have described the spectrum of these diseases. As their fibromyalgia reverses with guaifenesin, many children will require fewer dietary restrictions, and some will eventually need none at all. Others will have to avoid overconsumption and will ever be guided by their singular responses. We are sorry to report that only this hunting and pecking system with its adverse lapses will determine your child's ultimate diet.

> I started him on guaifenesin and the hypoglycemia diet. Within two weeks I had a different child. No problems with participation from him. He is so into this diet and treatment that he won't even cheat to have some pasta. If you need a child to be the spokesperson for this treatment he would be the one! We have taught a class on fibromyalgia reversal and mapping, he has been the pediatric case to practice mapping on. (This does cause him pain but Motrin works.)
>
> —*Kathie B., RN, CMT, northern California*

FOODS ARE OUR FUELS: A MORE DETAILED DESCRIPTION OF CARBOHYDRATE INTOLERANCE

> I had no difficulty following the diet, even though it was just before Christmas, and I was surrounded by sweets. It even seemed funny to me. When someone would offer me even the most tempting sweet I came to see before my eyes the witch offering Snow White the poisoned apple. Their protestations of, "Oh, one won't hurt, go ahead," came to sound like, "Wouldn't you love to have a headache? Please have one!"
>
> —*Cynthia C., East Lansing, Michigan*

Eighty-five to 90 percent of our foods are converted to energy, in the form of ATP. Almost all ingested sugars and complex carbohydrates are converted to glucose. Very little is needed for the construction of membranes and cell walls. A little is also hooked onto certain proteins including hormones to provide them their distinguishing characteristics.

As we have seen, each time we eat sweets or starches, insulin is released to drive glucose into cells, either for storage or to meet immediate energy demands. Through a series of biochemical steps, glucose is partly deposited as glycogen for future use or processed to ATP for sudden energy requirements. Because of their mass and working habits, muscles require huge amounts of both and take up about 80 percent of the carbohydrates that enter the body. The liver stores large amounts as glycogen but is less greedy in converting carbohydrates to ATP.

When there is an overabundance of fuel, the liver is assailed with external messages. Hormonal missiles bombard that organ and, consequently, its assorted enzymes explode into action. Insulin is the most significant of the released messengers, and it directs most of the ensuing activity. Under its direction, carbohydrate excesses are rapidly converted to glucose and strung together to create glycogen for future energy requirements. When it eventually fills the storage bins, leftover sugar is converted to fat, the lipids that are called triglycerides. They are exported into the bloodstream and, again under the auspices of insulin, taken up by adipose (fat) cells where they will reside until further instructed.

Much smaller amounts of insulin are needed for processing fats that are converted to fatty acids. Fat is also driven into other structures, particularly into muscles where certain of these fatty acids are readily used to make ATP. In fact, both heart and skeletal muscles prefer fatty acids as fuel. In the final analysis, it does not matter to mitochondria (the energy generators) whether it is fat or glucose that enters for processing. Both will be used mainly to make ATP or, in smaller amounts, building blocks for other requirements. Portions of our ingested fat, some 10 percent, can actually be converted to glucose.

Proteins are better used as building elements for a multitude of bodily structures. During digestion, they are broken down into amino acids, which are ultimately remade into other types of proteins. Amino acids are precious organic beads that go into making proteins, which are assembled with great precision like a string of pearls, using similar or dissimilar ones. The exact sequence is what makes each protein unique. The order in which they are strung is what characterizes each enzyme, many hormones, and other life-giving or protective chemicals that permit us to grow, repair, and develop immune systems. There is no life form without protein and its twenty component amino acids.

Proteins contain eleven amino acids that are each termed "essential," meaning that the body cannot manufacture them. They must be obtained from our diets. There are also two essential fats. The body can create all the energy it needs purely from fats and proteins. It may surprise you a bit but there are no essential sugars. We are quite capable of manufacturing any carbohydrate we might require for whatever purpose. The body may need carbohydrates to survive but we do not have to eat them.

In times of need, mitochondria can directly use certain proteins to make ATP. Amino acids therefore join the other two foodstuffs, carbohydrate and fat, as potential fuels. Fifty-six percent of these protein pieces can be converted to glucose, mainly by the liver and also, in appreciable amounts, by the kidneys. The process is called gluconeogenesis (the creation of new glucose). Clearly, whether we are fasting or eating a high-protein and high-fat diet, our body is assured of ample supplies of fuel as well as glucose.

This slightly technical discussion has been leading up to something. It should be apparent that we can quite safely pre-scribe a low-carbohydrate diet for children who have problems tolerating sugar. We are not advocating a no-carbohydrate diet. Our recommendations are for a balanced diet, one that simply avoids the wrong sugars and starches. Vegetables, dairy prod-ucts, and meats provide adequate amounts of minerals and vitamins and foster normal growth. As we will discuss shortly, leaner subjects must add sugar-free cereals or other grains and ample amounts of fruit to assure that they do not lose weight.

Correcting hyperactivity and hypoglycemia with a low-carbohydrate diet is perfectly healthy. In fact, it is mandatory. There are no deleterious effects on the young brain, liver, or kidneys. Your child's behavior will return to normal, some-thing you may not have seen recently. This will only happen as long as you maintain the necessary discipline to enforce the dietary corrections.

OBESITY

The worse I felt, the more determined I was to "eat right." And, of course, for my family to "eat right" so they would be healthy, too. The food pyramid with the big portion for grains and cereals at the bottom with eight servings a day was printed in every book I saw. So we switched to a diet rich in carbohydrates, and low in fat. I felt worse, and I gained weight. I was always hungry and faint. The more we adhered to the diet, the heavier we got. Cutting calories left us hungry and cranky. We thought we were doing everything right, but we did not feel well.

—*Cynthia C., East Lansing, Michigan*

As long as we are enjoining a battle with those attacking the safety of low-carbohydrate diets, we might as well go all the way. Let's briefly discuss the fattening of Americans, an accelerating process. Most of us are aware of the barrage by newspapers and newscasters concerning the epidemic of obesity in children and adults. Over 50 percent of adults in our society are overweight and almost 20 percent are grossly obese. Diabetes is at epidemic proportions in both children and adults. These numbers swell in certain ethnic groups. Statistics for children are rapidly approaching the horrifying numbers tabulated in adults. Type II diabetes, the kind usually known as "adult onset" and strongly linked to obesity, is now appearing in children across the country. Why on earth is this happening?

In our land of plenty we eat in abundance, more than enough at each meal, and we even snack in between. This unrestricted carbohydrate intake can cause problems for children, as it certainly does in adults. It should be clear to us all that our efficient storage system, designed to preserve the human race, is now responsible for the epidemic of obesity. Truthfully, both children and adults are being seriously infected with a very contagious virus described nicely by someone else as "affluenza."

We are told that the junk and fast foods are part of the problem. Added to that, television, video games, and the Internet are switching our kids from athletes to couch potatoes. The school system is decried for poorly enforcing gym and exercise class requirements. All this seems logical, but does it fully explain our expanding girth?

Remember our statement early in this chapter? There is only one hormone that can drive fat into fat cells: our storage hormone, insulin. It is willing and able to fill all of the warehouses within these adipose cells (adipocytes), spurred by the primal fear that today's feast may be our last. Insulin's purpose is to save for that rainy day that never comes in our excessively nourished society.

What are the components of our abundant meals and in-between snacks? Unfortunately, we rarely crave a slab of beef, a piece of chicken, a bucket of creamy butter, or a cup of olive oil. We eat those things as take-it-or-leave-it accompaniments to our mashed potatoes, crusty breads, and pasta. What would our slices of bread be like without sugared peanut butter, jelly, or jam? Pasta is "healthy" so we do it one better and eat it with sweetened tomato sauces. Salad dressings, even the oil and vinegar kinds, list corn syrup or dextrose on the label. What would a meal be without the dessert that follows? For snacks there are French fries, buttered popcorn, ice cream, doughnuts, candy, sugary snack bars, and an endless array of sweets. We wash all of them down with soda, lemonade, or chocolate milk—all sweetened. Even our so-called healthy snacks, such as yogurt and low-fat cold cuts, are laced with dextrose, honey, or corn syrup. The carbohydrate portions of fast food meals may be supersized and in turn supersize us, the consumers.

The sheer number of calories inherent in our carbohydrate-laden meals and snacks cannot be used for energy immediately. The body wastes nothing and therefore stores everything with food value. We have already seen that sugars and starches best stimulate insulin releases. Once surpluses are converted to fat, they are packaged into triglycerides (a troika of fatty acid molecules) for transport to the ever-hungry fat cells. We repeat: Insulin is the villain. It almost single-handedly triggers the enzymatic reactions that further swell our already excessive, chubby depots.

In urban mythology, ingested fat is usually blamed for making us obese. It seems logical to a layperson that fat equals fat. On television talk shows nutritionists slap down pounds of ugly lard to illustrate dramatically its nastiness. But in the absence of sugars, fat is not readily stored since there is only a meager release of insulin. The reality is that fatty acids (such as the stearic acid in beef) provide handy fuels for making the energizing ATP. That process is greatly accelerated when there is a relatively low supply of glucose. The heart and other muscles secure much of their energy by using stored fatty acids between meals and all night during sleep. Although the brain usually prefers glucose it will also use fatty acids for its energy requirements. We have already seen that certain portions of ingested fats (glycerol), along with some proteins, are converted to meet glucose needs, and no shortage develops even on very-low-carbohydrate diets.

We hope you have understood the thrust of our mini-biochemistry lesson. The summary is simple enough. Eating more fuel than we need for energy results in the carbohydrate portion being stored as fat. Insulin demands that fat cells accept the new fat whether or not they are already overly expanded. Low-carbohydrate diets safely permit weight reduction because protein and fats release much less insulin. In addition, protein and fats will be extensively burned as fuel and allow mobilization of fat deposits once insulin is no longer interfering.

This flies in the face of recent medical wisdom that suggests we should replace as much fat as possible with complex carbohydrates. Luckily, newer medical papers are finally challenging this poor advice. Many of us have stood on the sidelines even while advocating the benefits of a lower-carbohydrate diet to our heavier patients. I have done so for the past thirty-eight years, but now it is time to be more vociferous. Robert Atkins, M.D., a noted cardiologist who has written many books about low-carbohydrate diets, and several other dissenters have been correct all along.

Children and sweets should be hyphenated: They stick together throughout a youngster's life. To children, sweets are real food. Parents and other well-meaning adults are guilty of cultivating this relationship when they give sugary treats as a bribe or as a reward. Kids learn the drill and use it effectively from a very young age. Insulin is released each time carbohydrates are eaten, and genetically susceptible kids eventually deteriorate into symptomatic hypoglycemia.

Given this background, it is fair to wonder if it is possible for your hypoglycemic child to correct his antisocial behavior and, if overweight, lose pounds in the process. It is, but mainly through your efforts. Diets should be prescribed only for sound medical reasons, but as you have gathered, two of these are obesity and hypoglycemia. The necessary changes are safe and these diets still contain more than enough carbohydrates. We realize these restrictions will generate a battleground that tests your will against your child's demands. However, because these conditions are rapidly corrected in the young, your skirmishes should be brief. It does not take long for a child to realize he or she is feeling better. The older ones will actually relish being in control of both their emotions and their appearance.

> About a year ago we eliminated all sugar from Lance's diet because we noticed it caused his behavior to be much worse than merely "wound up." The only word that could adequately describe him is "belligerent." Even the no-sugar-added fruit juice was too much sugar for him. Dr. St. Amand suggested we might see further improvement if we would give the hypoglycemic diet a try. Since we are vegan, we wondered if that would even be possible. I have to tell you that we noticed such a huge difference within the first few days of the hypoglycemic diet that I can't imagine life without it. Lance is more calm, agreeable, and obedient.
>
> —*Cathy O., Bakersfield, California*

STRICT DIET FOR HYPOGLYCEMIA AND WEIGHT REDUCTION

Choose any foods from the following list.

Meats and Fish

All meats (most cold cuts contain sugars—check labels)
All fowl and game
All fish and shellfish

Dairy Products

Eggs, any style
Butter and margarine
Any natural cheese (bleu, Roquefort, cheddar, cream, Gouda, Swiss, etc.)
Cottage and ricotta—½ cup limit
Cream—heavy and sour

Fruits

Fresh coconut
Strawberries (limit 6–8 per day)
Avocado (limit ½ per day)
For flavoring:
Cantaloupe (limit ¼ per day)
Lime or lemon juices (limit 2 tsp. per day)

Vegetables

Asparagus
Bean sprouts
Broccoli
Cabbage (1 cup a day limit)
Cauliflower
Celery
Celery Root
Chard
Chicory
Chinese cabbage (limit 2 cups per day)
Chives
Cucumber
Daikon
Eggplant
Endive
Escarole
Tomatoes
Greens (mustard, beet)
Jicama
Kale
Leeks
Lettuce (any type)

Mushrooms (any type)
Okra
Olives
Parsley
Peppers (chile, green, yellow, red, etc.)
Pickles (dill or sour—limit 1)
Pimiento
Radicchio
Radish
Rhubarb
Sauerkraut
Scallions (green onions)
Spinach
Squash (yellow or summer)
String beans (yellow or green)
Snow peas
Tofu
Tomatoes
Water chestnuts
Watercress
Zucchini

Nuts (limit 12 per day)

Almonds
Brazil nuts
Butternuts
Filberts
Hazelnuts
Hickory nuts

Macadamia nuts
Pecans
Pistachios
Sunflower seeds (small handful)
Walnuts

Desserts

Sugar-free Jell-O
Custard (make with cream and artificial sweetener)

Drinks

Club soda
Diet sodas (no sugar, caffeine-free)
Coffee (for hypoglycemics, decaf only)
Tea (for hypoglycemics, weak tea only)

Condiments and Spices

All spices including seeds (fresh or dried)
All imitation flavorings
Horseradish
Oils (all types)
Vinegar (all types)
All of the following if they are sugar-free:
Salad dressings (check bottle labels)
Worcestershire sauce
Mayonnaise
Mustard
Ketchup
Sauces such as hollandaise (no corn starch)

Miscellaneous

All fats
Atkins and other low-carbohydrate protein snack bars and powders
Caviar
Unsweetened pork rinds or jerky

LIBERAL DIET FOR HYPOGLYCEMIA AND WEIGHT MAINTENANCE

Add these foods to the strict diet.

Fruits (limit 1 piece of fruit every four hours: no fruit juices)

Apples
Oranges
Apricots
Papaya
Blackberries (½ cup limit)
Peaches
Blueberries (½ cup limit)
Pears
Boysenberries
Plums
Casaba melon (1 wedge limit)

Raspberries
Grapefruit
Strawberries
Honeydew melon (1 wedge limit)
Tangerines
Lemons
Tomato juice
Limes
V8 juice
Nectarines

Vegetables

Artichokes
Peas
Beets
Pumpkin
Carrots
Squash, winter and spaghetti
Onions
Turnips

Nuts (no limit)

Cashews
Peanuts
Soya nuts

Milk and Desserts

Milk, whole, nonfat, low-fat, and buttermilk
Sugarless diet puddings (limit ½ cup a day)
Sugar-free ice cream (limit 1 cup)

Breads

Three slices a day of sugar-free white, whole wheat, sourdough, or
   light rye. No more than 2 slices at one time.

Miscellaneous

Carob powder
Puffed rice, shredded wheat, or other sugar-free cereals
Wheat germ
Brown or wild rice (limit 1 serving 3 times a day)
Flour, gluten or soya only
One cup popped popcorn
Gravy, made with gluten or soya flour only
Tacos, enchiladas, or corn tortillas (limit 2)
No sugar added preserves (limit 1 tablespoon)
Atkins and other low-carbohydrate snacks and bake mixes

Foods to Avoid Strictly

Dried fruits
Potatoes
Lentils, garbanzo, or lima beans
Corn
Refried or baked beans
Barley
Black-eyed peas (cowpeas)
Rice
Bananas
Pastas (all types)
Burritos and flour tortillas
Tamales
Sweets of any kind

Do not use products that contain dextrose, glucose, hexitol, maltose, sucrose, honey, fructose, corn syrup, or starch. NO CAFFEINE FOR HYPOGLYCEMICS. This means chocolate (sugar-free) must be limited to 1 ounce a serving, and sodas such as Diet Mountain Dew should not be consumed.

Chapter 7

❦

The Protocol:
A Quick-Reference Outline

Fifty percent of the patients I see tell me, "Oh, this is easy!"
The other 50 percent say, "This is very hard and complicated."
The answer lies somewhere between the two comments—it is
not easy, but it is easy enough to do if you want to get well.

—Claudia Marek

We hope our book is sufficiently straightforward to make it
possible for you to recognize fibromyalgia in your children. We
have asked you to digest a lot of information in the previous
chapters because there is a lot to learn and very little that is
tangible. The vagueness and all-pervasive symptoms of fibromyalgia make it difficult to fully visualize. Therefore, let's simplify your diagnostic chore in outline form.

Most of you reading this book are women who suffer from
fibromyalgia. However, you may not be the only faulty-gene
distributor in the family. If your child is very young, chances

are that both you and the father harbor either dominant or recessive genes for the disease. The individual or combined parental memories of childhood symptoms should alert you to the possibility that you have transmitted your legacy.

FIBROMYALGIA: MAKING THE DIAGNOSIS

The main reason I suspected fibromyalgia in Andrew was his leg pain at night, which started before he was two. There were occasional nights when he would awaken crying and parental comforting was inadequate to calm him. A dose of Advil and in twenty minutes or so he would go back to sleep for the night. When Andrew was four, I asked his pediatrician about these leg pains. His answer was that children need a reason to be crying in the night so they will say their stomach hurts, or this hurts, or that. I didn't argue at the time, but it didn't fit. I can tell the difference between a truly in-pain cry and a general "I don't know what I want" or "I don't want you to leave" cry. Ask any mother who has had a baby with an ear infection and she'll be able to tell you as well.

—*Holly S., Los Angeles, California*

Suspect fibromyalgia in children if they experience a number of the following list of common symptoms:

Younger Children

Doubling up and crying (this suggests abdominal pain)
Gas cramps without any obvious dietary connections

Constipation, seemingly without reason

Repeated bouts of diarrhea without infection

Urinary infections or strong urine odor or painful urination when there is no infection

Irritation of the vaginal lips and tissues deeper in the opening

Unexplained nighttime crying in obvious pain

Crying that cannot be consoled or pulling away when handled

Limping when walking

Skin irritations or rashes such as hives, eczema, tiny blisters, or pebbly bumps

Irritated or gunky eyes

Fatigue ending activities normally enjoyed and forcing rest periods

Older Children (basically any of the adult symptoms)

Fatigue or nonrestorative sleep

Irritability

Nervousness

Depression

Insomnia

Impaired memory and concentration (inattention)

Falling school grades

Anxiety

Salt or sugar craving

Sweating excessively or sudden flushing of the face, hands, or feet

Headaches

Dizziness (imbalance) or vertigo (spinning)

Blurred vision or irritated eyes

Nasal congestion

Bad breath and fleeting metallic tastes

Ear ringing or other transient sounds

Numbness or tingling fingers, toes, face
Restless legs, leg or foot cramps
Repeated bouts of nausea, gas, bloating, constipation, or diarrhea
Burning on urination or repeated bladder infections or strong urinary odor
Vaginal irritation
Brittle nails
Itching or rashes
Allergies
Excessive sensitivity to lights, sounds, or odors
Growing pains

> I am taking my son to see Dr. St. Amand because I've realized that he has complained of fatigue for years. But he has tried to hide it or live with it. When a teen boy goes out to buy vitamins, there is a hint. I now realize that he has complained about being tired in the morning for a long time. He seems only to get worse.
>
> —*Jayne C., San Diego, California*

Almost no one has all of the symptoms, especially at the same time. Adolescents have not lived long enough to amass all of an adult's complaints. In addition, the body is merciful and admits only so much pain. When one system is more intensely affected, the brain suppresses signals from other distressed organs or structures. Thus, severe headaches may block the perception of pain emanating from the legs, hip, or back. As malfunctioning intensifies in other areas, new symptoms may break through, seemingly wiping out the old ones. These variable, irregularly timed, and inexplicable complaints are exactly what should alert a discerning parent. The diagnosis should become more apparent with each successive cycle of symptoms. The sooner a parent can connect these individual attacks into a cohesive mesh, the sooner a reluctant physician may be urged to treat.

GUAIFENESIN PREPARATIONS AND DOSAGES

- Liquids with either 100 or 200 milligrams of guaifenesin per teaspoon (no prescription required). Sugar- and alcohol-free liquids are available, and certainly preferable.

- Tablets or capsules containing 200 to 400 milligrams of guaifenesin (no prescription required).

- Tablets containing 400, 600, or 1,200 milligrams of guaifenesin (prescription required).

Your child should be given pure guaifenesin in one of the above forms. Guaifenesin is without side effects, but commonly added compounds such as pseudoephedrine (a decongestant) and dextromethorphan (a cough suppressant) can cause problems. Such additives are not safe for the long-term treatment of fibromyalgia. They are certainly useful, however, for a limited time when they are needed during an acute illness. (Phenylproloanamine—PPA—also marketed in combination with guaifenesin, has recently been withdrawn from the market.)

I worked with "special children" before I had to abruptly end my nursing career due to FMS. . . . I encountered many challenges with children (three years to ten years old) and giving them medicine. The first thing to try is to crush the tablet or get the sprinkle or powder form, and put it in applesauce or pudding. . . . If this doesn't work, you can put it in "magic" Sprite and dissolve it. . . . This would work most of the time. You can do the same with the liquid. You can let them drink it with a straw, as a special treat, also. Capsules are often easier for children to swallow, and the texture and taste are better.

—Helen

FINDING YOUR CHILD'S DOSAGE

My parting words to you are that once you have established the dosage don't play around with it. Go through it, not around it. Watch like crazy every day for salicylates and believe that every day you are getting closer to a symptom-free existence. We do believe. We've seen evidence that is too strange to explain any other way.

—Nancy E., Dallas, Texas

Find a physician, massage therapist, physical therapist, or chiropractor to examine and map your child before starting guaifenesin. Sufficient sites should be sought to provide a reasonably representative set of lesions so that you have a baseline for future and serial comparisons.

Begin at 300 milligrams of guaifenesin twice a day (every twelve hours). If your child's symptoms get distinctly worse, that is probably the correct dosage. Hold there. After one month your child should be remapped to confirm the efficacy of the current dosage. Mapping frequency after that time should be determined by how well your child feels. As long as progress is being made, you do not need to change the dose. *If your child is improving on 300 milligrams twice daily, you may skip to the next section.*

If your child feels no worsening of symptoms after one week, raise the dose to 600 milligrams twice a day. Remap after one month at this level. If he or she feels no difference and the map shows no improvement at this time, increase the guaifenesin to 1,800 milligrams a day. (A single tablet may be taken either morning or night and two tablets at one time on the alternate dose; one tablet three times a day is equally effective.) If, after another month, no changes are apparent either by observing the child or upon mapping, dosage requirements may be even higher (applies to 10 percent of patients only). Before raising the dosage, recheck all products for any source of salicylates. This small investment of time is mandatory, because if its receptors are blocked, no amount of guaifenesin will benefit your child.

CHILDREN'S PRODUCTS THAT OFTEN CONTAIN SALICYLATES

We cannot emphasize enough that failure to remove salicylates from your child's products will block all benefit from guaifenesin. You must teach your child to rigorously avoid salicylates, both synthetic (salicylic acid) and natural (oils, gels, and extracts with plant names). They must be totally avoided whether they are contained in medicinal oral compounds (aspirin, Pepto-Bismol, herbal remedies) or in topical products. This includes mouthwashes, as well as herbal candies or breath fresheners. Young children use only a few items, making control fairly easy. With teenagers, especially girls, this proves a difficult task that requires constant vigilance.

The most common salicylates children encounter:

- Pain medications (both topical and oral) such as aspirin, Ben Gay, and Aspercreme.

- Medications for upset stomach, such as Alka Seltzer and Pepto-Bismol.

- Medications for topical ailments: Wart removal compounds and dandruff or medicated shampoos frequently contain salicylic acid. Cortisone and burn creams sometimes add aloe. Products for sore throat or sore mouth (for example, Aspergum) or those with plant oils such as clove or eucalyptus will block guaifenesin. Other products similar to Vicks rub and cough drops contain menthol or mentholatum and are therefore prohibited.

- Herbal medications: No supplements with a plant name (such as echinacea) can be used. A dictionary helps to decipher botanical names. In addition, bioflavonoids or herbs (for example rose hips or alfalfa) are often added to vitamins and deliver salicylates.

- Sunscreens often include salicylate components (octyl salicylate or octisalate) or aloe.

- Shampoos, conditioners, and soaps: Many have plant additives. Fragrances are not a problem unless your child is sensitive to them.

- Baby wipes and washes: Watch out for added aloe.

- Toothpastes and mouthwashes: Most mouthwashes and toothpastes contain members of the mint family and often added salicylic acid (Listerine, Scope). Bubble gum, cinnamon, and fruit flavors are acceptable if they do not also contain mint, like Children's Colgate or Oral B.

- Gum and breath mints: Avoid mint, peppermint, spearmint, or wintergreen oils (synthetic or natural).

For older children, in addition to the above:

- Topical medicinal products such as acne lotions or solutions often contain salicylic acid or plant compounds such as witch hazel, arnica, camphor, or menthol.

- Deodorants may contain castor oil or aloe.

- Shaving items: Lotions, creams, and gels should be checked for aloe, mint, menthol, or mentholatum. Vitamin E, baby oil, and lanolin are acceptable. Do not use razors that add an aloe strip adjacent to the cutting edge. Teflon moisturizing strips or vitamin E are safe.

- Skin care products: Facial scrubs or toners for oily skin may contain witch hazel, menthol, or salicylic acid. Liquid soaps frequently contain plant oils or aloe. Lotions and bubble bath preparations must be carefully scrutinized for botanicals such as almond oil, cucumber extract, rose oil, sandalwood, lavender, or any other so-called aromatic herbs.

- Cosmetics: Check carefully for salicylic acid and any plant derivatives. Foundations and lipsticks frequently include plant oils such as castor, camphor, and jojoba or the popular aloe. Bronzing creams and sunless tanning agents may also include the bark extract bisabol. (Powders and powder eye shadows are usually safer bets than liquids.) Waxes, acids, and distilled inorganic chemicals, though sometimes extracted from plants, are not blockers.

- Nail products: Like the ends of the hair, nails are dead and do not transfer substances into the bloodstream. Small cuts and tears in the cuticles could potentially absorb aloe or castor oil that sometimes appears in nail polishes or polish removers. These tiny amounts will not usually block, but why risk it?

A list of salicylate-free products appears on our website, *www.fibromyalgiatreatment.com*. It is by no means a complete listing of acceptable products but was written to serve as a shopping aid only. When using our list or any other, it is absolutely necessary to check each product label every time you shop, because manufacturers make frequent changes without notice.

WHEN TO SUSPECT CARBOHYDRATE INTOLERANCE OR HYPOGLYCEMIA

The diagnosis is not easily made in younger children. Hyperactivity and aggressive behavior are the only reliable clues. The uncontrollable child who can be calmed within five minutes by eating a jam and peanut butter sandwich is a strong suspect. If eating sweets or heavy starches converts your child into a wild and untamable creature within an hour or more, you have added evidence. The clincher comes when feeding your child causes his or her behavior to improve. These simple observations are all the clues you will probably find to lead you to the diagnosis of carbohydrate intolerance (hypoglycemia) in a very young child. Sugar and sweets will cause disruptive behavior, eating again will calm it.

The older the child, the more likely carbohydrate intolerance symptoms will mimic the adult form. A five-hour glucose tolerance test is punitive and somewhat brutal. It is also not very accurate. Avoid it, and use your observational evidence to make the diagnosis. Any of the following may be noted when hungry:

Hand tremors
Irritability
Severe fatigue
Sweating or clamminess
Heart pounding
Frontal headache
Anxiety or panic attacks

MAKING THE NECESSARY DIETARY CORRECTIONS

Bouts of low blood sugar, hypoglycemia, and obesity are hardly expressions of optimal health. Dietary changes are mandatory. If a child has fibroglycemia, guaifenesin will reverse the fibromyalgia portion but it will not alter the carbohydrate-induced symptoms without dietary changes. If a child is obese, poor conditioning may blunt subjective improvement. However, please remember no diet is necessary for treating fibromyalgia.

For Obesity with or Without Hypoglycemia/Carbohydrate Intolerance (Strict Diet)

The low-carbohydrate diet must be observed as written with no substitutions permitted. Children will lose weight and correct hypoglycemia (carbohydrate intolerance) despite eating as much as they desire from the following list. Once weight goals have been achieved, or if no weight loss is necessary, foods from the subsequent list—the Liberal Diet—must be added.

- Meats: all meats, including poultry, red meat, pork, and lamb; all fish and shellfish; cold cuts must be checked to insure that no sugars have been added.

- Dairy products: sour cream, heavy whipping cream, margarine, butter, and other vegetable oil spreads are acceptable. All natural cheeses are allowed—½ cup per day limit on cottage cheese and whole milk ricotta cheese. (No processed cheeses such as American are permitted.)

- Fruits: fresh coconut, avocado (½ per day limit), cantaloupe (¼ per day), strawberries (6–8 per day). Two teaspoons of juice from lemons or limes may be used each day.

- Vegetables: All of the following are acceptable: asparagus, bean sprouts, broccoli, brussels sprouts, cabbage, cauliflower, celery, chard, chicory, Chinese cabbage, chives, cucumber, daikon, eggplant, endive, escarole, greens (dandelion, mustard, beet), jicama, kale, leeks, lettuce, mushrooms, okra, olives, parsley, peppers (red, green, yellow, hot, etc.), pickles (dill, sour—one per day), pimiento, radicchio, radish, rhubarb, salad greens, sauerkraut, scallions, snow peas, spinach, string beans (green or yellow), summer squash (crook-neck, yellow, patty pan, zucchini), tomatoes, water chestnuts, watercress.

- Nuts (limit 12 per day): almonds, Brazil nuts, butternuts, filberts, hazelnuts, hickory, macadamia nuts, pecans, pistachios, walnuts, or a small handful of sunflower seeds.

- Desserts: sugar-free Jell-O, custard (made with cream and artificial sweeteners), cheesecake (no crust) made with cream cheese, sour cream and artificial sweetener or sucralose (Splenda).

- Beverages: artificially sweetened drinks from mixes such as Crystal Light, Country Time, or Kool-Aid made with sucralose. Club soda, sugar-free flavored soda waters, beverages made with zero-carbohydrate syrups such as Da Vinci. Caffeine-free diet sodas.

- Condiments: all sugar-free sauces, such as hollandaise, Worcestershire, ketchup, mayonnaise, and soy sauce. All herbs and spices, such as dill, horseradish, basil, and oregano. Imitation flavorings and any type of oil and vinegar are acceptable as long as they are sugar-free.

Parents may want their children to eat foods lower in saturated fats and higher in oleic acid (such as olive oil). If so, fatty cold cuts are to be avoided, and visible fat should be trimmed from meat to avoid cholesterol. Foods may be grilled, broiled, or baked to avoid frying unless the so-called safe oils (olive, safflower, canola, corn, peanut) are used and not overheated. Solid margarines are best replaced by liquid ones (avoid trans and use cis oils, if they are labeled). Nuts are lower in fat when they are dry-roasted.

Diet to Control Hypoglycemia and Maintain Weight (Liberal Diet)

If your child is of normal weight, but has symptoms of hypoglycemia, the following foods should be added to those on the strict diet. It is important that the youngster adds the allowable carbohydrates in the restricted amounts and types listed here (for example, three slices of sugar-free bread a day). If insufficient carbohydrates are consumed, your child will lose weight and may find it difficult to regain it. Like the strict diet, this must be followed as it is written for the first month in order to control the symptoms and allow healing.

Foods allowed in addition to those listed above on the strict diet:

- Fruit: 1 piece of fruit every 4 hours, V8 juice or tomato juice. Blackberries and blueberries are limited to a single ½ cup serving every 4 hours. Casaba and honeydew melons are limited to 1 wedge every 4 hours.

- Vegetables: Artichokes, beets, carrots, onions, peas, pumpkin, winter/spaghetti squash, and turnips.

- Nuts: Quantity limitation is removed. Add cashews, peanuts, and soy nuts. Your child may have sugar-free peanut butter and other nut butters with a small serving of sugar-free jelly.

- Dairy products: Whole, low-fat, nonfat milk, or buttermilk. Unsweetened (or artificially sweetened) yogurt. Small servings of no-sugar-added ice creams or frozen yogurts are okay.

- Breads and cereals: 3 slices of sugar-free bread daily, no more than 2 slices at one time. Sugar-free flat breads and cracker-breads such as Wasa, 3 servings per day, with no more than 2 at one time. Sugar-free cereals such as puffed wheat, puffed rice, and shredded wheat are well tolerated. One cup of popcorn (popped) is also allowed. Brown or wild rice may be eaten, one serving each meal.

- Desserts: Sugar-free diet puddings (½ cup a day), cookies and muffins made with low-carbohydrate bake mixes. One serving of no-sugar-added ice cream.

- Miscellaneous: Carob powder, flour (gluten or soy only), wheat germ, 2 corn tortillas such as in 2 tacos or 2 enchiladas.

In time you and your child will both learn how many carbohydrates can be consumed without feeling any ill effects. It is a hunt-and-peck system that may allow resurgence of hypoglycemia if tested with too much carbohydrate or too often.

We hope you realize by now that your child's treatment does not lie in your physician's hands only. It is a deeply shared responsibility. Doctors do not have the time or willingness to stay abreast of manufacturing whims. It would be unrealistic to expect them to conduct a review of all of your children's products. Physicians cannot monitor your child's diet on a daily basis. All chronic illnesses require lifestyle changes, and fibromyalgia and fibroglycemia are definitely no exceptions.

> I renewed my efforts to communicate my desperation to my doctors, but all they had to offer were antidepressants or a blood pressure medication known to cause depression. The same questions I had had since childhood continued to prey on me: Why was I different? Why could I not just get up and be like everyone else? I felt isolated by my pain, unable to even begin to communicate to anyone what my life was like, and increasingly devastated and guilty from the effect my pain was having on my family.
>
> —*Cynthia C., East Lansing, Michigan*

During the time your children are under treatment, you have a chance to teach them as much as possible about fibromyalgia. It is a wonderful opportunity to learn the cause of their symptoms and how the medication reverses the illness. Some of this comprehension will persist as children grow older. At some point—usually in their teens—they inevitably stop taking guaifenesin out of either defiance or denial. Symptoms

will gradually return when treatment is neglected or abandoned, and these attacks will eventually provide ample reminders that faulty genes eventually prevail. Most young
adults will willingly resume treatment when they start to feel
worse. Our support will help to protect them from the dis-
tressing years that many of us have known.

Chapter 8

Helping Your Children
with the Reversal

I've developed some pretty strong opinions on how children are treated in our society. Their complaints are often not taken as seriously as are those of adults, and they're not allowed to speak up for themselves. We who understand what children with FMS are experiencing must become their advocates. To test my theories as to how children and young adults are treated I tried an experiment a few years ago. I was going back to college . . . and I decided to tackle my childhood nemeses, piano and physical education. . . . I briefly explained my illness and then tackled the classes within my own limitations. Far from being picked on, I was singled out as an example. . . . What a boost to my self-esteem! However, several freshmen in my classes who may have had limitations of their own but did not know how to speak about them were treated less admirably. In piano class I explained to my instructor that I needed to have a few minutes for stretching exercises before I could sit down at the piano and that I could not play for more than twenty minutes without getting up to stretch. Again, I became the star pupil while younger students were accused of being lazy and not practicing enough. I do not mean to imply that all the young people who had problems in those classes suffered from FMS. I don't know what their limitations were. But, because of their youth and inexperience in standing up for themselves, those who may have had limitations were perceived in exactly the same way as those who really weren't trying.

—*Lou, Clemmons, North Carolina*

We hope the previous chapters have taught you how fibromyalgia manifests in children. We tried to instruct you concerning its devastating effects on body and brain functions. Though the exact chemistry is not known, we trust you understand something about guaifenesin and how it initiates reversal by overcoming a defect that we hypothesize exists within certain kidney cells. We have expressed how crucial it is that you fully grasp the significance of salicylate block. We trust you are prepared to replace products with safe counterparts.

We think this chapter should be equally helpful. It is concerned with the navigational skills you may need to steer your child and his or her peers and instructors through the unpredictable waters of a changeable illness. Your aim, obviously, is to restore the special exuberance that is the right of every child. The task now at hand is to think about what you can do to help while you are both waiting for your child's symptoms to clear.

No youngster wants to be different or become identified

with an illness. However, if your child learns he or she can monopolize your soothing attention by being sick, his or her attitude will reflect that, and little games will begin. The world hardly needs another manipulative individual who copes only by inflicting miseries on self and family. It is therefore all the more important that you attack the disease early, well before abnormal behavior is ingrained. You should nurture and comfort but only for the purpose of creating an individual who is healthy, happy, and productive. It is not too much to ask that one should mature, unafraid to fully explore all talents and proclivities. After all, isn't this why you are considering guaifenesin treatment in the first place?

> When everyone else would take part in PE with enthusiasm, I could barely do the things required of me. I always wondered how others could do the things they did because I was sure that everyone had to feel as bad as I did. I didn't know that I wasn't the norm. . . . My stomach kept me in the bathroom for much of my young life!
> —*Cristy T., Little Rock, Arkansas*

BEGINNING TREATMENT

I never quite had the stamina other children have. I was an active child, able to play, but also very exhausted afterward, and it was extremely difficult to keep up. Climbing stairs was an effort due to the pain in the back of calves. I recall, as a teenager, dancing was an effort, and I would try to find excuses to speak to people rather than dance. I traveled with a singing group and what should have been an excellent experience turned into one that was exhausting. When I would have down days people thought I was lazy. There were peaks and valleys with my level of ability to function as a teenager. I learned how to work quickly when I could. . . . My brother and sister used to make fun of me when I didn't have the strength to do the things they could do. My mother would accuse me of simply not wanting to do it. Nothing could be further from the truth.

—*Linda B.*

With the youngest children there is little to explain, because they cannot grasp very much. If they are inquisitive and raise questions about certain symptoms, limit your answers to those issues. Keep your chat matter-of-fact and add that you have a good medicine that takes care of such problems. Though it doesn't work overnight, their symptoms, such as sore legs, won't continue much longer. As children grow older, you may infuse greater detail when they probe more deeply. You might point out that all kids have differences. Some wear glasses, some are small, and some have to be very careful in the sun because they burn too easily. There may be an acquaintance who must be treated for diabetes or friends who require other medications. During the course of every discussion, please stress that there will be no lasting restrictions on what they can do—fibromyalgia isn't that kind of illness.

Early on, you should instruct them that they must avoid putting certain things on their skin or into their mouths. Sunscreens are a good point of departure to introduce the concept of salicylate blocking, even if you do not use that name. With such examples, children can be taught that certain products will absorb through the skin and totally stop their medication from working. Provide children with special places for their personal products such as toothpaste, shampoo, body lotion, and the sundry things adolescent girls eventually use. This will reinforce the importance you attach to choosing safe products.

Planning for younger children is simple, as there are no concerns about adversely affecting schoolwork during the early cycles of reversal. When they are tired or cranky they can rest. When they don't feel well for a few days, handle each cycle as you would any other illness. Treat the symptoms while waiting for the good days lying just ahead. When they are generally achy, provide relief with pediatric Advil or Tylenol. Warm baths and rubdowns greatly soothe stiffness and soreness. We doubt any of us has forgotten the therapeutic value of a parent's touch.

While providing comfort, reassure them and yourself that cycles are brief in children and improvement is rapid. Stress that they are normal kids and their sickness is only temporary. To that end, they should be allowed to play soccer, swim, or participate in any of the activities they especially enjoy. They will actually feel better, because the tight tissues loosen up during the course of play.

If a young child requires dietary changes for hypoglycemia, control is relatively easy. He or she is under the supervision of a responsible adult during all the waking hours. If you point out the bad effects of sugar, even very young children quickly accept that, though very tasty, it is what makes them aggressive, hyperactive, and generally out of sorts. If they are able to articulate their feelings, they may even comment that they can't help acting as they do at certain times. They quickly grasp that cranky and unreasonable behavior chases everyone away, even a loving parent.

The connection with nontolerated foods is best made as soon as the attack is over. This is a wonderful time to reinforce your previous warnings about the adverse behavioral effects of certain carbohydrates. Timely reminders of how much better they feel and act when eating correctly eventually teach children to avoid offending sugars and starches on their own. Parents are always amazed at how quickly children understand this. Just reinforce the positive by an outpouring of attention and praise when they spontaneously eat the way they should. Compliment them on their wonderful new perception and mature behavior.

Unfortunately, children act like adults. They too are human, and from time to time will yield to temptation. After they make the inevitable mistakes, discuss the cause and effect and then drop the subject. It is very important that you avoid punitive actions, since negative reinforcement is not the greatest teacher. Just feeling sick and out of control and sensing your disappointment usually are sufficient punishment.

Provide several copies of the list of foods your hypoglycemic child should avoid. Post one on the refrigerator for baby-sitters and visiting relatives to use for reference. Hand them to the adults in day-care and preschool centers. Put another in your child's backpack and stress that it is there to be shared with anyone who should be aware of restrictions. In this day and age this will not seem unique, since many children have allergies and also carry lists to school. Be alert to inadvertent errors, such as automatically giving kids apple juice or other sweets at day care and camp. Tell the persons in charge about such pitfalls. Also arm your child with sugar-free drinks, water, and safe snacks. A properly cultivated habit can easily be continued throughout the school years, including the days of field trips, or camp-outs.

> One of the hardest things is that my son and two nieces have this, too. . . . He has the stiff neck and shoulders, pal-pable lumps, the same jerking as he drops off to sleep that I have, a constant postnasal drip, the acute sense of smell and sensitivity to light and sounds, sore knees and legs, irritable bowel symptoms, and depression. He acknowledges it and is going to start the guai. My two nieces don't even want to hear the word. One of them has said, "I'm never gonna get that disease, you used to DO things and I'm never gonna be like you!"
>
> —*Jane B., Clarendon, Pennsylvania*

Older children with fibromyalgia already know they are not like all other kids. Many have learned to mask odd feelings and sensations. They long ago learned to make excuses, be-cause they couldn't tolerate being sick or different. If you have fibromyalgia and they have witnessed your suffering over the years, they will most assuredly not want to have what you have. Many will state it point-blank: "I don't have what you've got."

We think it useful advice when dealing with older children to concentrate on what problems they admit to and avoid comparing them to you or some other relative. Speak specifi-cally about their own fatigue, headaches, cognitive or intesti-nal problems—not yours. Ask them if they would like to try some medicine for a while, one that should make them better. Don't scare them off with tales of what will probably happen if they don't take guaifenesin. Just explain it matter-of-factly and be realistic. If your child is in denial, you won't get any worthwhile cooperation pushing some strange medicine to be taken twice a day while simultaneously giving up a bunch of favorite products. It would be better to request a fair trial and specify some finite period of commitment. You could request a pledge for a bona fide, six-month attempt. If you get no interest the first time you broach the subject, try again during the next bad cycle. Skip drama and scolding by gently pointing out symptoms that may be eliminated. Eventually, when your child is ready, he or she will take you up on your offer and accept help.

> As a child I remember my mom saying, "Teri was born tired," which makes me realize that even then I was experiencing the fatigue that is associated with FMS. When I was in grade school I lived about half a mile or so from school. I used to bribe one of my friends to carry my heavy school bag home for me. I realize now more than ever that perhaps I have no idea what it's like to experience the energy that most people take for granted.
>
> —*Teri, Coventry, Rhode Island*

It is worth remembering that children may not perceive themselves as you do. If the illness appeared before memory set in, a child has no way of realizing that it isn't normal to wake up exhausted after sleeping all night. There is no basis for knowing that aches and cramps in their legs aren't growing pains and shouldn't be there. They may have no concept of what it is like to feel great.

> After being on guaifenesin for several months, my son con-
> fided in me that his legs used to ache terribly when he went
> up the stairs at his high school. When I asked him why he
> didn't tell me he said, "I thought it was normal." He then
> asked if I remembered him complaining when he was little
> about his legs hurting and being tired when I took him
> shopping. Yes, I did remember that, but thought it was the
> complaints of a little boy who hated to shop. If only I could
> have known and understood then.
>
> —*Nadine T., Delaware*

While collecting stories for this book, we discovered that half of the youngsters with whom we spoke thought all children were tired and achy. They actually wondered how other kids were tough and brave enough to keep functioning despite pain and fatigue. Many of the others realized they were different from their friends and described their struggle to hide their secret. It takes a lot of patience and reinforcement to get such children to verbalize symptoms and emotions. If they already see themselves as having a defective character trait, such as laziness, as opposed to having an illness, it is the responsibility of both parent and physician to teach otherwise. It is as much part of the process as adding guaifenesin for reversal.

> My mother took me to our family doctor, who thought it
> was absurd that a child was complaining of pain. He told
> my mother that I needed to run and play more. In my

child's mind I took his comments to mean that I was lazy and not quite normal so I vowed to stop telling anyone about the pain. . . . And then there was my piano teacher. She would tell me that I had so much talent if I would just loosen up my shoulders and arms and let the music flow. . . . I would cry and continue to play, still feeling that I wasn't good enough and I wasn't trying hard enough. How much easier it would have been for us both if she and I could have understood that I couldn't loosen my shoulder.

—*Lou, Clemmons, North Carolina*

The avoidance of salicylates poses a variable problem. With younger children it's less of an issue because you are the one who buys their products. Instruct your older child, especially a daughter, that most products list ingredients. Also teach that a few things such as toothpaste do not have to describe all of the contents. A good rule of thumb for all teenagers and especially those with fibromyalgia is that they shop only in stores with a favorable return policy.

Unless they are already badly affected by fibromyalgia, it is sometimes a wiser plan to schedule when you begin their treatment with guaifenesin. This especially applies to older children, such as those in junior or senior high school. Difficult material is presented at these levels and grades may affect subsequent promotions more acutely. It is not so worrisome with the younger students since they will easily catch up. Ideally, guaifenesin should be initiated at the beginning of school vacations or in the less-demanding time of the early school year. Certainly avoid starting a few weeks before a tough exam or finals. It is easier on both parent and child to begin when schedules are less hectic and during less-demanding times when resting will be possible.

> I started them on the guaifenesin on June 3, 2000 (as soon as school was out). On three hundred milligrams twice a day, K., eleven years old, had more fatigue and more back pain. Not intolerable, but enough to make her take a nap several days. . . . She asked for Tylenol for all-over body aches and a headache. On three hundred milligrams twice a day, A., eight years old, had leg pains nightly, again controlled with Tylenol. She sometimes has leg pains in the daytime as well.
>
> —*Kathy, Atlanta, Georgia*

Since the first two or three reversal cycles may be arduous, allow your child a break from extracurricular activities such as music lessons or sports if he or she requests it. The need for such a hiatus naturally depends on individual stamina and the severity of the illness, as well as your child's own character. Reassure your child that he or she is actually beginning the process of getting well and a break is available if needed. Promise a quick resumption of the normal routine. Children should return to activities one by one without waiting to get totally well. They cope quite well even when they are only partially better. It is important they not feel they are missing out and that they remain active and involved with their peers.

> I can sit back and look at my childhood now and understand why I felt so different, like an outcast in a strange sort of way. I always had a lot of friends, but I knew deep down inside

there was something different about me. When I would talk about aches and pains they would call me a wimp, like nothing ever hurt them. As I got older, I couldn't do a lot of the physical activities that my friends could. I tried different sports but I was never good at any of them. I fatigued easily and was always getting injured, and I had this constant pain on my right side when I did anything strenuous. I was always the kid who was picked last for team sports.

—*Donna, Lomita, California*

Putting older children on the diet, if they are hypoglycemic, is more difficult because much of the food they consume each day is beyond your control. One hopes that instructions you give during vacations, weekends, and communal meals will have their impact. They will be reinforced by the deleterious effects that cheating produces with the resurgent symptoms it metes out in hard-to-forget lessons. Older children have the same symptoms as adults do. They'll experience the shaking tremor, the headaches, sweating, and the anxiety and pounding heart of hypoglycemia. Though they may not say so, you can be sure they are secretly vowing to themselves to avoid feeling like this ever again. You may not even have to point out the difference in their entire demeanor when they are adhering to their diet. Their friends may do this for you!

RELIEVING YOUR CHILD'S SYMPTOMS

My eleven-year-old daughter began having headaches at age eight, then neck and shoulder pains. We saw every doctor imaginable . . . no cause could be determined. Kidney-draining homeopathic drops helped a little but didn't last. . . . We had a mouth splint made because someone thought this was TMJ. We took her off all sugar products for six months. We treated her pains with Tylenol. . . . I am so relieved now to have a reason for my daughter's complaints. Doctors have accused me of anything and everything. Drugs prescribed have been of *no* help and were often harmful. I knew my daughters were not crazy. I knew I wasn't crazy.

—*Kathy, Atlanta, Georgia*

Like adults, children have varying sensory thresholds, including the tolerance for pain. Some children will experience severe pain with fibromyalgia, others will merely complain of stiffness and display some lack of stamina. For others, "fibro-fog" will be the greatest problem, and many will suffer the embarrassment of the irritable bowel syndrome. It is almost certain that after they begin guaifenesin, their symptoms will initially worsen. Unlike adults, children will have only a few months or years of illness to reverse. Therefore, cycles do not last long and purging is rapid.

Acetaminophen (Tylenol) or nonsteroidal anti-inflammatory medications (Advil, Aleve, ibuprofen, and so forth) are usually sufficiently effective. If necessary, combinations of the two may be used, since each works on pain somewhat differently. For occasional relief of restless sleep, children's Benadryl may be used. It has the advantage of not being habit-forming but may induce next-day somnolence. There are also over-the-counter preparations to help with the irritable bowel and other symptoms, but enlist your doctor's help, as not everything may be appropriate for your child. Always bear in mind that it is not possible to relieve all pain and discomfort of fibromyalgia. Just remaining active and involved is of great solace for older children. Their overwhelming desire to be with friends often provides all the encouragement needed.

We cannot speak out adamantly enough against using strong medications on children or adolescents. We have already seen far too many who have ended up as quasi-invalids, not because of their fibromyalgia but from the horrors of habituating drugs. Parents sometimes vicariously suffer their child's pain and become overprotective. They will occasionally even demand of their physicians that narcotics be given for pain and sedatives for sleep. As their children build up drug tolerance, parents become desperate and embark upon the search for even stronger drugs. The demand leads to heavier-duty drugs in addictive combinations in an attempt to totally relieve all symptoms. As symptoms eventually break through each drug in turn, parents inadvertently enclose their child within a circle without end, one that includes dependency and possibly lifelong habituation.

The side effects of sleeping pills and narcotics take a huge toll on children's lives. Their acuity is dulled, they have daytime fatigue, and as a result may miss many days of school. As such times accumulate, children fall farther behind, become isolated, and eventually can no longer catch up. They are soon stigmatized by their failures and newly acquired "dummy" status. Their inability to participate in extracurricular activities deprives them of a normal childhood and crucial social interaction and development. If they are given antidepressants, their highs and lows are eased, but they are also deprived of the chance to fully experience their emotions. Though it may not be politically correct to say so, mind-altering drugs are mind-altering drugs, whether acquired from a well-meaning doctor or from the drug dealer down the street. Any parent considering narcotics, hypnotics, muscle relaxants, or the like for a child should take a long, hard look at the consequences and ask if there is an alternative.

> My daughter was officially diagnosed yesterday with FM by a pediatric specialist. This doctor told me there wasn't much she could do but put her on Zoloft, and then she told me how sorry she was. However, I did tell her about the guai, and she told me to go for it. . . . This specialist is a young, open-minded pediatrician and is sort of interested in this protocol although she had never heard of it. . . . My daughter is eleven and tells me she is very sad that she has this disease. It breaks my heart.
>
> —*Darlene S.*

We understand your desire to help your child. Both of us have children with fibromyalgia and have watched them suffer. But we ask that you believe us. We have seen and experienced too much to remain silent. The truth is that less is more when it comes to children. The less fuss, the less medication, the better. Children are wonderfully strong and resilient, and with a little support and understanding they will quickly heal.

She was not like my two other children, who ran and played all day long. She would always be sitting on the sidelines watching or "holding other people's things for them." She started to complain of constant neck and shoulder pain. We bought every herbal remedy under the sun for her. . . . We tried everything but nothing consistently worked. We watched a very profound change in her from when she was eleven through thirteen. She became very foggy in her mind, could not remember the math she had done the day before. She also got discouraged, and every day became a "burden" to her that she felt was becoming too great to bear. . . . We started her on guaifenesin . . . and soon she was sleeping and kept telling me how different she felt. She was able to do her schoolwork and *remember* what she had learned. She was running with other kids and not getting tired. She has days of cycling when she hurts more than others, but they seem to pass quickly. Her depression is a thing of the past, which has been the best blessing of all.

—*Wendy M., California*

SCHOOL

During my son's high-school years he seemed to work harder than most for his grades. Some days he would come home, stomp up to his room, and shout, "I know I have ADD," or, "I am learning disabled." He started taking guaifenesin in the spring before he went to college the following fall. His first-semester grades in college were all A's and one B. The fog had lifted.

—*Nadine T., Delaware*

All but the youngest children attend school, and that institution holds an important place in your child's life. Even if your child is too young for grades "to count" for college, how he or she achieves affects how he or she will perceive him- or herself. How he or she manages those early years will have a great influence on expectations and lifelong performance. Failures make wonderful teachers but too many can be burdensome and will only prove beneficial when offset by successes.

Although he has always managed to be athletic, and do it very well, it always seemed as though he was not as agile physically nor had the same endurance as others. I thought it would be interesting to have him mapped and see if his stiff neck and various aches and pains went beyond the norm. I was right on! His map was full. It is only looking back and realizing all the symptoms of FMS that it all makes sense now. . . . As he headed into puberty he was constantly hurting, much more than his fellow athletes. Of course his complaining was never accepted by coaches and players alike. And then came the fatigue. I know boys are tired a lot when they are growing, but this just seemed more extreme than most. He actually fell asleep at volleyball practice when he was a freshman in high school. The coach sent him home. Fortunately, he was an understanding person. Other symptoms he has had are impaired concentration, sweating, headaches, dizziness, restless legs, itching, rashes, and even a bladder infection as a young boy. . . . He still suffers some pains but overall is able to compete on a college volleyball team, go to college, work, participate in a fraternity and various other activities at school. . . . He has the energy to keep going. I am so grateful to have started him early in his life so his reversal has been much easier and quicker than mine.

—*Lori R., Irvine, California*

As the parent of a child who may need a little extra help, it's up to you to make his or her needs known clearly and succinctly. Of course, you will also have to work within the limitations imposed by the situation. With perseverance and more than a little prodding, you can set your child up to succeed in his or her world. A tough start doesn't spell disaster, not if you remain firm in the expectation that your child do his or her personal best. You will get cooperation if you persist, because there are caring teachers and physicians who are prepared to work for your praiseworthy goals. After all, this is your child and there is not much room for compromise.

One of the first moves in helping schoolchildren is to set up a conference with each teacher. Delay is dangerous, because it will eventually become an unavoidable meeting, one held too late to change opinions. Too many absences and poor grades and too much inattentive behavior may have already convinced some teachers that your child is an underachiever. The simple tactic of using an early approach and explanation will make a big difference. Ask for enough time so that you may speak with the appropriate teachers in detail. Have an outline and a list of the things you need to remember. Try not to overwhelm the teacher with a ream of paper and medical records. From experience, we can tell you that the more succinct the material you provide, the better the chances it will be read. Everyone is busy, and your child's teacher is no exception.

Explain that your child has fibromyalgia, and if that draws a blank look, you can try chronic fatigue. A short letter from a physician might be in order, since teachers may not know much about the disease. They may know enough to link fibromyalgia with pain, but understanding fibrofog, cycles, and irritable bowel is too much to expect. Emphasize that symptoms come and go and most of the time there will be no need for special help or attention. See what the teacher offers. There are often many options available if they are discussed or requested in advance. For example, with a doctor's note most schools allow extra time for standardized tests, and work can be done on computers if your child has problems writing. Go to the meeting prepared with a list of ideas that you think will help your child get his or her work done within whatever boundaries you feel are reasonable.

If the teacher seems unwilling to work with you, don't hesitate to visit a principal, vice principal, or counselor. Most school boards have a whole hierarchy of supervisors who can help. Luckily, in this age of disability awareness and legally mandated equal access to education, the consciousness of most administrators is fairly high, but be prepared to stand your ground. There are many programs available to children whose parents take the time to pursue them.

The best thing for everyone involved is to understand that you have high expectations for your child. At the same time, you must be realistic about his or her limitations. Tell teachers how often you think your youngster will need to rest during otherwise mandatory phys ed classes or how often he or she might have to miss school altogether. Don't expect schools to allow your child to skip PE for the entire year, and please don't even wish that for your child. You should desire as much total participation as possible. Without special testing that reveals disability, schools cannot waive all the mandated requirements regarding attendance and performance. Putting your child through the process of being declared disabled may do far more harm than good, so that course should be carefully weighed when it comes to fibromyalgia, which will resolve if treated.

Most of all, the point of meeting the teacher, who spends so much time with your child, is to establish communication. Descriptions of fibromyalgia should be accurate to help establish your credibility. Teachers may feel encouraged to give your child a little leeway simply by the facts you present. This will be especially true if your child displays an acceptable level of performance most of the time. Be realistic and don't expect to achieve all of your goals in one session. Make sure teachers feel welcome to call you to share observations and express concerns. This would be the best of all microworlds for you, the student, and schooling. It will not always spin as you desire, but recall that we offer this counsel only as a temporary measure. Organized planning is meritorious and far better than just producing patchwork results. You are reading this book not merely to cope with a bad situation but to enrich a young life with the full vigor it deserves.

Epilogue

We began this book with the story of a laggard lamb that could not run as the other lambs did. All I could tell by observing her was that she was different from the others, though she tried hard to be like them and join their games. We will never know what prevented her from playing with the others.

Our fibromyalgic children seem different when we watch them in the company of their peers. As observers, we can only look for clues, watch and listen carefully. When we have seen and heard enough, it becomes our duty to help. We must articulate their pains, fatigue, and cognitive impairments when they can't and, above all, find them help. If they are older, we must listen to their complaints and take them seriously when others, who do not know them as we do, do not.

For some of us, reading this book will awaken memories long dormant. Our own childhood sequences may now be buried within the heap of far more flagrant adult attacks. Recalling these symptoms becomes even more poignant when we are faced with our own children suffering as we have. Our emotions are very often deepened by our own guilt, knowing that our children have inherited this illness from us.

But we must look deeper. Properly handled, fibromyalgia can be safely and readily controlled, ultimately making it almost a nondisease. The ease of recovery will reassure our children, so that they, in turn, will not be intimidated at similar prospects in their own progeny. (Perhaps we can even convince them that this may be the worst of their genetic legacy and how wonderful is the remainder of the genetic pool we have bestowed upon them!)

We have written this book to brighten what has been bleak. Too many parents have escorted their children from doctor to doctor, more frustrated with each opinion and each specialist. Savings accounts are drained, precious time is wasted, and children remain in pain and exhausted. Too many children have grown up despondent about being different, as though the illness were somehow their fault. By early adulthood, the impression has been instilled in them that they suffer from defective character traits rather than a treatable condition.

We have come, through our experiences, to urge a slightly militant stance. Parents must be prepared to assault their children's physician with evidence. The possibility of fibromyalgia, once raised, greatly facilitates its affirmation. Parents should be ready with an outline of their own history, especially that of their youth. When faced with the similarities in an organized fashion, the pediatrician or family doctor will more deeply reflect on the information and data being presented.

Even with the diagnosis in hand, parents must still find a

doctor to treat their youngsters rather than merely attempt to relieve their symptoms. Too often, physicians think nothing of giving a child an antidepressant or muscle relaxant. They will, however, balk at writing a prescription for guaifenesin "because it is not for fibromyalgia" or "it hasn't been proven yet." Double-blind studies will one day provide the final proof. Meanwhile, we cannot wait in silence and simply wallow in double-blind-itis. We need an urgent solution. It is proper to ask doctors about the safety of guaifenesin compared with any of the utterly unsafe alternatives they have suggested. We assure you that no medication has been marketed "for fibromyalgia." Some compounds have been shown to relieve some symptoms in an unimpressive percentage of patients— that is the best that can be said of any of them.

We once tagged our protocol as "not for the faint of heart," but then neither is it pleasant being the parent of a sick and miserable child. This situation is even less tolerable once we learn that an effective treatment exists. It is safe, affordable, and can be prescribed by any licensed physician. We must be firmly determined if we are to get our children successfully diagnosed and treated. We must persist until all of us with fibromyalgia are well. All of us have the right to a full life and liberty from pain. The pursuit of happiness is a moral and inalienable right we deserve for ourselves and may then assure for our children.

Resources

For More Reading about Fibromyalgia

Marek, Claudia. *A Patient Expert Walks You Through Everything You Need to Learn and Do the First Year: Fibromyalgia, an Essential Guide for the Newly Diagnosed.* Marlow & Co., 2002.

St. Amand, R. Paul, and Marek, Claudia Craig. *What Your Doctor May Not Tell You about Fibromyalgia.* New York: Warner Books, 1999. Contains in-depth information about the theory behind the guaifenesin protocol, etc. Website has handouts for interested physicians, etc. *www.guaidoc.com.*

Starlanyl, Devin J., and Copeland, Mary Ellen. *Fibromyalgia and Chronic Myofascial Pain Syndrome.* Oakland: New Harbinger Publications, 1996 (second edition published 2001). Has a chapter on pediatric fibromyalgia.

Starlanyl, Devin J., and Copeland, Mary Ellen. *The Fibromyalgia Advocate: Getting the Support You Need to Cope with Fibromyalgia.* Oakland: New Harbinger Publications, 1998. Her website has additional material: *www.sover.net/~devstar.*

Williamson, Miryam Erlich. *Fibromyalgia: A Comprehensive Approach.* Walker and Co., 1996. (Contains a chapter about children and FM, including those on guaifenesin.)

Williamson, Miryam Erlich. *The Fibromyalgia Relief Book.* Walker and Co., 1998.

Williamson, Miryam Erlich. *Blood Sugar Blues: Overcoming the Hidden Dangers of Insulin Resistance.* Walker and Co., 2001 (Foreword by R. Paul St. Amand, M.D.).

Diagnosing Fibromyalgia and Treating with Guaifenesin

Videotapes are available from: The Fibromyalgia Treatment Center, Inc., Post Office Box 7223, Santa Monica, CA 90406. Order forms at *www.fibromyalgiatreatment.com.*

Videotape 1: *Treatment and Mapping.* This tape includes Dr. St. Amand explaining the illness theory and protocol to a new patient and has a demonstration of the mapping technique. $20.00.

Videotape 2: *Mapping Demonstration Only.* This tape is for interested practitioners, and is $10.00.

Please see the website for shipping and handling, or include $3.95 per item. All proceeds from these tapes are given directly to the nonprofit foundation for fibromyalgia research. Please allow three weeks for delivery.

Canada: In Canada books, tapes, and toothpastes can be ordered (along with other resources) from Julie at *www.fibronorth.com.*

Great Britain: *www.ukfibromyalgia.com* has a guaifenesin resource section and some information.

Salicylate-Free Products

Personal Basics by Andrea Rose: salicylate-free and fragrance-free skin care and hair care products and lipsticks. Also a high-quality sunscreen and tartar control toothpaste (vanilla flavor). Andrea is a fibromyalgic who is dedicated to creating quality products for others on guaifenesin. Call 877-712-ROSE for a brochure, or go to *www.andrearose.com*. Her products will always be salicylate-free.

Grace Dental Products: Dr. Flora Stay, D.D.S., and her husband, Andy, have made a variety of dentrifice products for patients using guaifenesin. Her toothpastes are baking-soda-based, and flavored with xylitol. (FibroSmile tastes like traditional toothpaste, but there are many other flavors children will like as well.) Also mouthwash. Grace Products, 178 S. Victoria Ave., Suite A, Ventura, CA 93003. Telephone: 805-981-2986. They do not test on animals, and donate 10 percent of profits to homeless and abused children. You can also order from their website: *www.drstay.com*.

Illuminare Cosmetics: excellent-quality cosmetics, all salicylate-free, and the best-quality sunscreen with good SPF coverage. Owner Ruthie Molloy has a sister on guaifenesin and is eager to help us. She is located in Folsom, California, and can be reached at *ruthie@illuminarecosmetics.com*. Phone (toll free) 866-984-0877. Ruthie will provide samples for a nominal charge. Website: *www.illuminarecosmetics.com*.

Paula's Choice: Our favorite cosmetic critic, Paula Begoun, has a special section on her website listing the products in the line she's created that don't contain salicylates. (Not all of her products are salicylate-free, but those that are, are marked carefully.) Her staff will answer your questions truthfully and will contact us with questions if they can't answer yours. Telephone 800-831-4088. Paula's Choice, 13075 Gateway Drive, Suite 160, Seattle, WA 98168. Website: *www.paulaschoice.com.*

Tom's of Maine: Tom and Kate Chappell have two toothpastes that can be safely used with our protocol. These are the strawberry and orange-mango flavors. These are sold in stores around the country. Information is also available from the company at *www.tomsofmaine.com.,* or by calling 1-800 FOR TOMS, Canada 207-785-2944.

Books for Product Reference

Begoun, Paula: *Don't Go to the Cosmetic Counter Without Me.* Updated regularly, currently fifth edition. Seattle, WA: Beginning Press. Website: *www.cosmeticscop.com.* Also has a newsletter by subscription. An excellent article by Paula Begoun called "Face Facts" can be found at *www.stretcher.com.stories.* Don't take your daughter to the store without reading it!

Winter, Ruth, M.S.: *The Concise Dictionary of Cosmetic Ingredients,* fourth edition. New York: Crown, 1994. Ruth Winter also has a website and a free newsletter at *www.brainbody.com.* This book is a good purchase (it's paperback and will fit in a purse or backpack) for teenage girls who want to try new products constantly. It lists all cosmetic ingredients in a dictionary format and can be used to instantly check the salicylate status of products. Also updated regularly.

Websites to Help with Product Concerns

Product list put together by Claudia Marek: *www.fibromyalgiatreat-ment.com.*

Product list put together by Tesa Marcon and the guai-support group: *www.netromall.com/guai-support.* Also has a list of chemicals that can and can't be used as well as plant names and products. Has international products, especially from Australia and the United Kingdom.

Other lists exist elsewhere on the Internet. All lists, including the above, should be used as **guidelines only.** Products change daily and need to be rechecked each and every time they're purchased.

Shopping for Products Online

Browsing for products or buying them online is an excellent option, especially if you live in an area where some products may be difficult to find. Almost all companies have their own sites, which you can find easily via a Web search or by using the name (for example: bonnebell.com).

www.drugstore.com (which also links to beauty.com) has good prices and won't charge shipping if you order a certain amount. This site sells all sorts of beauty products, as well as such things as sunscreens, deodorants, supplements, and hair products. The advantage to this site is that the ingredients are listed, and you can check products carefully before you buy. The type is large enough to read, and you don't have to run all over town. They have a liberal return policy and make it easy for you to do so if you don't like what you've ordered for any reason.

www.sav-ondrugs.com also sells many products, with ingredients listed.

www.sephora.com sells high-end products, many of which have listed ingredients.

www.gloss.com has a huge inventory of products but does not list ingredients. You'd have to do your homework before you purchased here.

www.dermatik.com has products for acne and so forth. All are salicylate-free.

Many other stores have online shops now, including Target, Wal-Mart, Nieman Marcus, and Macy's. Some include ingredient listings and some don't. If your daughter has a favorite line she can look at these and other sites. Also, all companies have a contact-us button on their sites to request information.

Resources for the Diets

Please note that most low-carbohydrate books are designed for weight loss. Please review recipes carefully to make sure they do not conflict with the hypoglycemia diet.

Books

Atkins, Robert C. (M.D.). *Dr. Atkins' New Diet Revolution*. Evans and Co., 1992.

Atkins, Veronica C., and Atkins, Robert C. (M.D.). *Dr. Atkins' Quick and Easy New Diet Cookbook*. Fireside, 1997.

Gassenheimer, Linda. *Low-Carb Meals in Minutes*. Bay Books, 2000.

Heller, Richard F. (Ph.D.), and Heller, Rachael F. (Ph.D.). *Carbohydrate-Addicted Kids: Help Your Child or Teen Break Free of Junk Food and Sugar.* Dutton, 1998.

Heller, Richard F. (M.D.), and Heller, Rachael F. (M.D.). *The Carbohydrate Addict's Cookbook: 250 All-New Low-Carb Recipes That Will Cut Your Cravings and Keep You Slim for Life.* Dutton, 2000.

McCullough, Frances Monson. *The Low Carb Cookbook.* Hyperion, 1997.

McCullough, Frances Monson. *Living Low-Carb. Hyperion,* 2000.

And one more, because it's so good, and an absolutely necessary resource if you have diabetes in your family:

Bernstein, Richard (M.D.). *Dr. Bernstein's Diabetes Solution.* Little, Brown and Co., 1997. website: *www.normalsugars.com.*

Diet Resource Websites

www.atkinsdiet.com. Dr. Atkins's website has information from his books, scientific papers, and newsletters.

www.grossweb.com/asdlc. Website for the low-carb support group. This site has links to many shops, cookbooks, and so forth, and is an excellent place to start. If you join the group beware of two things: This is a weight-loss-oriented group, and the volume of posts is very high.

www.immuneweb.org/lowcarb. Vegetarian low-carb website, helpful especially if you have a daughter (or son) who is flirting with the idea of becoming or is a vegetarian. Great resource for vegetarians who suffer from hypoglycemia.

Low-Carbohydrate Shopping Sites

www.atkinscenter.com. The Atkins Diet website homepage. This site offers many resources for low-carbohydrate dieting, including many recipes and products such as mixes, shakes, and snack bars.

www.eas.com. EAS products, including shakes, bars, et cetera. Telephone 877-971-0947.

www.cest-bon.com. C'est Bon offers a few cookbooks and several recipe ideas.

www.latortillafactory.com. Low-carbohydrate tortillas (which can be ordered in bulk and frozen). Telephone 800-446-1516.

www.low-carb.com/low-carb. Many products, including ketchup, sauces, BBQ sauce, and syrups.

www.lowcarbchocolates.com. Selection of sugar-free candy bars.

www.lowcarbohydrate.com. Protein crunch cereal, energy snack mixes, and protein bars. Good resources for school lunches and traveling.

www.davincigourmet.com. Sugar-free syrups made with Splenda for beverages, cooking, and so forth.

www.sugarlessshop.com. 1 Stop Sugarless Shop contains an online catalogue, which offers many low-carb products. It also has a database of sweetener names with descriptions.

www.specialcheese.com. Snacks and chips made from pure cheese. Telephone 800-367-1711.

www.sugarfreemarket.com. Offers a wide array of low-carb and zero-carb products "from soup to socks."

www.sugarfreeparadise.com. More products, including bagels, brownies, and crackers. This site also carries kosher products.

www.thinner.com. Includes a recipe database, "Carb Counter," discussion group, and links to new low-carb products.

Pediatric Pain/FMS Resources

Since this book is intended for young people, it's time to say a word about the Internet. Most of our children, by the time they're old enough to want to communicate with their peers, know their way around a computer and e-mail. (I was recently shocked to get an instant message from my niece Camilla, who is still in elementary school!) Computers are especially good for children who may feel isolated by their illness. As research tools they can be invaluable if your child doesn't feel up to going to the library, or if the family needs additional support or resources.

If you don't have a computer, consider purchasing one. Newer models coming out for Internet access and simple word processing will be inexpensive. Your child won't need all the latest gizmos to write to pen pals or join a support group.

A simple search on google.com or any other search engine will turn up websites about kids and chronic illness or pain. Many offer the option to e-mail others, or to find a "pen pal." Here are a few that seem excellent.

www.faculty.fairfield.edu/fleitas/contents.html. Website called Bandages and Blackboards for children of all ages. Has pictures, stories, and pen pal areas. Many teens and younger children have posted their stories. Set up by Joan Fleitas, Ed.D., RN, at Fairfield University in Fairfield, Connecticut.

http://pages.prodigy.net/turnip/childrenandteens.html. Children, teens, and young adults, sourcebook for teachers, attending school with FMS and educational rights for young persons with FMS/CFIDS are a few of the resources here. Also carries "Fibromyalgia/CFIDS and Children" by Gretchen Parker, an excellent article.

http://members.aol.com/fibroworld/juvFM.html. For those on AOL has links to other sites.

http://home.bluecrab.org/~health/sickids.html. Links to other sites and many personal pages and stories.

www.cfids.org/youth. CFIDS Organization of America has a place to sign up for pen pals, a chat room, and other discussions.

Support Groups/Sites for Fibromyalgia Symptoms

Interstitial Cystitis/Irritable Bladder

The IC Network, 707-538-9442. Jill Osborne, Founder. 4773 Sonoma Highway, Santa Rosa, CA 95409. Website: *www.sonic.net/jill/icnet/welcome/html.*

Interstitial Cystitis Association, 212-979-6057 (has a section on girls). PO Box 1553, Madison Square Station, New York, NY

10159. Website: *www.ichelp.com.* 120 S. Spaulding Drive #210, Beverly Hills, CA 90212.

Vulvar Pain/Vulvodynia

National Vulvodynia Association, 301-299-0775. PO Box 4991, Silver Spring, MD 20914-4491. Website: *www.nva.org.*

The Vulvar Pain Foundation, 335-226-0704. Joanne Yount, Director. PO Box Drawer 177, Graham, NC 27253. Website: *www.vulvarpainfoundation.org.*

Also: *www.vulvarhealth.org* has an area for girls, as does *www.wdxcyber.com/vulva.html.*

Irritable Bowel

Irritable Bowel Association, 1440 Whalley Ave. #145, New Haven, CT 06515. Website: *www.ibsassociation.org.*

Information page: irritable bowel in children: *http://niddk.nih.gov/health/digest/summary/ibskids.*

Book: Van Vorous, Heather. *A Patient Expert Walks You Through Everything You Need to Learn and Do: The First Year, IBS: an Essential Guide for the Newly Diagnosed.* Marlow & Co., 2001. Heather van Vorous had IBS as a child, and several other children's stories are included in this book.

There are also some websites that offer support information, including *www.parentsplace.com,* which has information on a variety of symptoms in children.

Miscellaneous Contacts

Americans with Disabilities Hotline: 800-446-4232 or 800-949-4232.

The United States Department of Justice Resource Page for Disability Law: *www.usdoj.gov/crt/ada/cguide.html.*

National Clearinghouse for Women and Girls with Disabilities. Education Equity Concepts, Inc., 114 East 32rd Street, New York, NY 10016. Phone: 212-725-1803.

Index

lumps:
   and helping your children with
      reversal, 126
   pediatric FM diagnosis and,
      44–45
   as pediatric FM symptom, 23, 38

mapping, 87–88
   case studies on, 15, 84, 136
   in FM diagnosis, 12–13
   guaifenesin and, 109
   and helping your children with
      reversal, 136
   in pediatric FM diagnosis, 42–45,
      50, 87
   pediatric FM symptoms and, 27
   pediatric FM treatment and, 45,
      48, 50
   salicylates and, 65
   tips on, 44–45
margarine, 97, 116
mascaras, 76
massages, 38, 124
meats:
   in hypoglycemia and weight
      reduction diets, 97, 114, 116
   nutrition and, 91, 93–94
medical histories:
   in FM diagnosis, 11–13
   pediatric FM symptoms and,
      38–39
medications, 13, 51–55, 142
   addictiveness of, 133
   case studies on, 38, 107–8, 118,
      134–35
   dosages of, 43

for FM in women, x–xi
for FM symptoms, 11
FM treatment and, 53–54
for gout, 52–53
and helping your children with
     reversal, 121–24, 126–30,
     132–35
pediatric FM diagnosis and, 43
pediatric FM symptoms and, 27,
     31, 36, 38
salicylates in, 63–64, 66–73, 76,
     110–11
side effects of, 118, 133
and theory of cause of FM, 55
see also guaifenesin
memory impairment:
   as FM symptom, 6
   nutrition and, 82, 86
   pediatric FM diagnosis and, 44,
      105
   as pediatric FM symptom, 24
menthol, 71–73, 110–11
milk, 93, 101, 114, 117
mind-altering drugs, 134
mineral oils, 71, 76
mint, 62, 66, 70–73, 111
mitochondria, 57, 90
Motrin, 66, 88
mouthwashes, 64, 67, 69, 72,
     110–11
muscle relaxants, 134, 142
muscles, 18
   in definition of FM, 1–2
   FM diagnosis and, 12
   FM symptoms and, 6
   FM treatment and, 53

About the Authors

R. PAUL ST. AMAND, M.D., is a graduate of Tufts University School of Medicine. He has been on the teaching staff at the Los Angeles Harbor/UCLA Hospital, Department of Endocrinology, for over forty-three years. He is currently an assistant clinical professor at the UCLA School of Medicine. Dr. St. Amand discovered guaifenesin's use as a treatment for fibromyalgia, and his work is cited wherever the substance is mentioned.

CLAUDIA CRAIG MAREK, M.A., is a medical assistant tutored, trained, and taught on the job by Dr. St. Amand. She has cowritten medical papers with Dr. St. Amand and has counseled fibromyalgia patients for more than ten years.

R. PAUL ST. AMAND, M.D., and CLAUDIA CRAIG MAREK are authors of *What Your Doctor May Not Tell You about Fibromyalgia*.

WHAT YOUR DOCTOR MAY *NOT* TELL YOU ABOUT FIBROMYALGIA

The Revolutionary Treatment That Can
Reverse the Disease

by R. Paul St. Amand, M.D., and
Claudia Craig Marek

In this innovative book, Dr. St. Amand, the country's foremost expert on this subject and a former sufferer of fibromyalgia, presents his amazing discoveries based on forty years of research. This book offers the first effective protocol for reversing fibromyalgia: a program that uses guaifenesin, an inexpensive, proven-safe medication available from your doctor. This is the definitive guide to this troubling, often misdiagnosed disease.

"Groundbreaking. . . . Dr. St. Amand's research will permit fibromyalgia to become merely a memory."

—Dr. John Willems, M.D., head, Division of
Obstetrics and Gynecology, Scripps Clinic

more . . .

WHAT YOUR DOCTOR MAY *NOT* TELL YOU ABOUT CHILDREN'S VACCINATIONS

Hidden Dangers, Pros and Cons, and Safety Measures That Can Protect Your Child

by Stephanie Cave, M.D., F.A.A.F.P., with Deborah Mitchell

Vaccines used to be considered a godsend. Today there are troubling signs that we may be *over*-vaccinating our children—sometimes with alarming repercussions. Dr. Stephanie Cave, an expert in the field of pediatric inoculations, gives parents information they need to make informed, responsible choices. Based on the most recent research, this guide explains different vaccinations and offers a blueprint for which ones are safest and when to give them.

"A must-read . . . an important resource. . . . Dr. Cave's tips on reducing vaccine risks will save lives."

—Barbara Loe Fisher, cofounder and president, National Vaccine Information Center